INTENSIVE CARE

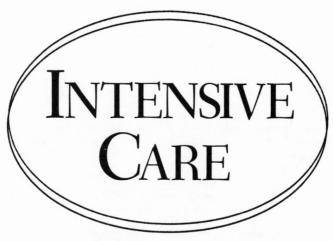

INTENSIVE CARE

A Family Love Story

MARY-LOU WEISMAN

Random House New York

Library of Congress Cataloging in Publication Data
Weisman, Mary-Lou.
Intensive care.
1. Muscular dystrophy in children—Patients—United States—Biogra-
phy. 2. Weisman, Peter, 1964–1980.
I. Title.
RJ482.D9W44   618.92'34   85-502
ISBN 0-394-52348-2   AACR2

Manufactured in the United States of America
24689753
First Edition

For Larry and Adam

The beauty of the world . . . has two edges, one of laughter, one of anguish, cutting the heart asunder.
—Virginia Woolf, *A Room of One's Own*

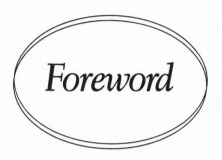

Foreword

Intensive Care is a love story. It is about the kind of love that knows no conditions, has no expectations and makes no demands. Most people lavish such love temporarily on babies, but few adults can give it to children or to one another. It is an archetypal love for which we all, whether or not we have ever experienced its sweetness, share a kind of collective nostalgia. That is the kind of love that my family had somehow to generate when we learned that our second son, Peter, had muscular dystrophy. This is the story of the love we gave and failed to give to one another and how Peter taught us to insist upon it.

It is a true story. I wrote it more like a novel than a memoir because I believed that the novel form would put me at a sufficient distance from my own situation to enable me to describe how life changes and what life feels like when it is lived with the full knowledge of death.

I did not want to limit what I had to say to the sad story of a dying child. Such a narrow focus not only limits, it distorts. After all, while Peter was dying, he was living. So, in fact, are we all. He was an entire person—funny, annoying, perceptive, original, stubborn—who went to school, rode a bike, talked dirty, and got into trouble. He was not just a doomed child. And those of us who loved him and cared for him were whole people too—cynical, angry, lively, naïve, and sometimes cowardly—who went to work, had friends, made love and paid bills. We were not just tragic figures.

I was interested in seeing what kind of reality might emerge if I could look at myself, my family and others as characters with the vivacity and purpose of actors in a drama, but a drama fabricated from the data of our lives, and told from my point of view. To that end, while I was writing the book, I gave us fictional names, hoping thereby to pull a fast one on myself, to watch myself, as if from a distance, if only for a moment. That magic moment, however brief, would give me the opportunity to walk around myself, to see myself as a three-dimensional stranger before I would inevitably recognize myself, break the spell and return to the one-dimensionality of self-consciousness. When I finished the book early in 1982 I went through the manuscript and gave us back our real names. The effect was like that of a zoom lens focusing in: sudden, drastic and alarming.

The characters in the book bear their actual names with only a few exceptions. Dr. Braverman is a composite figure representing a number of pediatricians who attended Peter. Drs. Kittenplan and Tierney preferred pseudoanonymity. Both have, however, read the manuscript as it relates to their roles, and have affirmed its accuracy. The names of certain minor characters in the hospital (Crystal Bocanfusco and Mr. Wisznicki) and at the Esalen Institute (Bernice, Claude, Felicity Plum, Dan and Molly) have been fictionalized but are based upon real characters and events.

The dialogue, with one exception, is based upon memory, notes from a journal that I began in 1971, and the recall of those friends and family with whom the conversations took place. After much consultation ("I'm sure I never said 'boob,'" my friend Sara Duskin advised. "I'd have said 'bosom'; *you'd* have said 'boob'") I hope that something close to what actually was said emerges.

The only exception is Peter. I began to take notes on his conversation as early as 1971—at first casually, in my journal. Then, when I started writing this book in July of 1978, when Peter was thirteen years old, I began to transcribe his words more scrupulously. All of Peter's significant dialogue is verbatim.

I would like to thank the members of my family and all the other people, some friends, some near strangers, who appear without fictional cover as characters in this book. To allow me to portray them as I saw them demonstrates an ego-defying integrity and generosity of spirit for which I am most grateful.

I also appreciate the help of Fredi Laporte, Verita Rickards, Dr. Kurt Hirschhorn, Dr. Lewis P. Rowland and Dr. John R. Iacovino in the verification of facts and preparation of the manuscript.

Finally, and most especially, I would like to thank my husband, Larry Weisman, and my aunt, Lily Harmon. I believe the book is better, and I, measurably saner, for their wise counsel and loving encouragement.

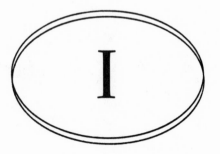

I

"Mommy! Mommy! *Mommy!*" The intercom on the bedroom wall pours Peter's waking voice into my dreaming ear. I am awake. My heart pounds. I taste tin in the back of my mouth. Before I know my name or where I am, or why, I reach for my throat in the dark and begin to undo the buttons of my nightgown, until I remember that mother's milk is not what's called for. Pete needs to be turned. It is the second time in one night. It's getting worse.

"Coming . . ." I depress the "talk" lever and whisper into the white plastic box. It emits a harrowing electronic squawk, reminding me that "talk" is broken; only "listen" works.

My husband, Larry, groans, rolls over in his sleep and grabs at the covers.

It's not so bad when I'm standing. Straining through the dark, frowning, hands stretched out in front of me, I know that when I feel the rug begin to end under the small, timid steps my bare feet are taking, my hands will touch the door that leads to the hall. I am learning my way in the dark. Walk a little too much to the left, and I collide with the bookcase; a little too far to the right, and I walk into the night table and the lamp falls over.

This time, one hand encounters the familiar feel of the fluting on the doorjamb; the other lands on the knob.

I am in the hall. I close the bedroom door and flick on the hall light.

Through the bathroom is the easiest way into Peter's room.

"Coming," I call softly, entering the bathroom from the hall. I remember to reach for the urinal lying on the back of the toilet. Maybe he has to pee.

"What is it, Pockie?" I bend over him, whispering so my voice over the intercom won't wake up Larry, but I hope it does. "What's the matter, Fudgetickle?"

"Turn me. I want to go on my side," Pete murmurs throatily, trying to stay asleep.

Side is the hardest. "I just moved you from your side to your back a couple of hours ago. Are you sure you want to switch back?"

"I'm sure," he says hoarsely.

"Okay, sweetie," I whisper.

In response, a phalanx of murderous feelings topple over in my chest, like so many ritual suicides. "You just stay nice and sleepy. Mommy will make you comfortable. Do you want to piss first?"

"I don't know if I have to," says Pete. "I'll try."

I tuck the plastic urinal between his legs, leaning down hard against the handle, pressing the bottom into the mattress to get the proper angle. With my left hand I lift his penis over the lip.

"Let me hold it," he says.

I take a spare pillow and tuck it under his arm, elevating it so that the geometry is just right and Pete can use two fingers to hold down his penis.

I press down; he holds. Nothing happens.

"It's going to come," he says. "I can tell."

"Don't worry," I reassure him, my right wrist beginning to ache with strain. It is dark, so I can grit my teeth.

"Here it comes," he announces. I feel the tiny stream of warm urine spend itself against the inside of the urinal neck. "That's all," he says.

I pull the urinal away and blot the tip of his penis with a tissue. "I'll go dump it," I say, moving toward the bathroom.

I worry as I pour and flush no more than four tablespoons of urine down the toilet whether Peter is losing control of his bladder, or whether he is merely growing more anxious, or whether maybe it's me who's anxious. I return to the bedroom to turn him.

Slowly I pull out the pillow that is tucked under his knees, allowing them to rest bent while he is sleeping on his back, and let it drop onto the floor near my feet. With the pillow gone, his legs fall open against the sheet, rotating outward from the hip. I slip my left hand between his head and the pillow, and exert all the pressure I can with my palm, upward against the nape of his neck, to lift his head enough to slide out the pillow smoothly. His head is the heaviest part of him. I feel the effort in the muscles of my belly, which tighten and tremble. I let that pillow fall to the floor.

White against white he lies, his limbs askew, where they have fallen, each weighted by its own helplessness, like objects spilled from a box. I bend to kiss his bellybutton.

"Over we go!" I whisper as I place one hand on each hip and flip him deftly onto his side. The rest of his body follows and resettles rakishly—legs scissored, one arm pinned under his side. The other arm, turned outward and extended, the elbow balancing on the elevated hipbone, waves faintly, eerily, in an involuntary gesture. I hasten to rearrange his disordered body into a model of innocent repose, tucking his lamb's-wool hippopotamus, Soft Gray, in the crook of his arm and the tips of his fingers under the corner of the pillow.

"Move my top leg forward," he mumbles. "That's good."

"Are you comfy now?"

"Yank my left arm down, just a little. Down and to the right." The left arm and shoulder are the trickiest. "That's good."

"G'night, Poindexter Bluntwhistle Flutter Pop McGee," I say, kissing the top of his shoulder.

"G'night," he answers. "Is the intercom on?"

"Yes, it is."

"Is the volume turned way up?"

"Yes, it is."

He cannot hear my bare toes tapping on the floor. His growing inventory of anxieties makes me impatient, and sad. But he hears it in my voice. "Because it took you a long time to come when I called you before. I called six times."

I can feel his helplessness, six times over, calling, then waiting, then calling in the dark. "I only heard the last two times, Pocket. I'm sorry. Sometimes I'm just sleeping so deeply that it takes a few calls to wake me up."

"I'm not angry." Peter protects my feelings better than his own.

"Are you all set now?"

"Remember to pull the sheet up over my head." I pull the sheet up as far as I can stand to, leaving the top of his head exposed. "Pull it up all the way over my head," he instructs. "I don't want to see the dark."

"Good night, Petie. I love you."

"Good night, Mommy. I love you too."

I pull his bedroom door closed behind me. I decide to leave the door between the bathroom and the hall open, just in case the intercom should fail. I'd have a better chance of hearing him through two doors instead of three. And then I know it doesn't matter. The roiling in my stomach and the panic in my brain tell me I'm not going to be able to sleep any more tonight.

I look down the hall toward the kitchen. Nice. Three rush chairs tucked under a pine table—one for Mommy Mary-Lou Bear, one for Daddy Larry Bear, one for little Adam Bear, and an empty space where the leaf extends and Peter's wheelchair fits under. A little desk in the corner full of cookbooks, pencils and a pale-green decorator telephone with a thirteen-foot-long rubber-coated spiral extension cord uncoiling toward the floor. The cord is singed black and melted to the wire in places where it has touched a red-hot burner from my efforts to talk and cook dinner at the same time. Above the desk, a bulletin board is paved with good intentions: Shakespeare at Stratford; yoga classes at the Westport "Y." I recognize it, but is it my life? Insomniacs are aliens.

I'll have a bowl of cornflakes, I decide, and make myself at home. But I eat it at the counter, hastily.

I wander into the living room and flick on the light. The living room surprises me. Lovely! Like a Dutch still life. The tables with their rich patinas, the antique opulence of lustrous brass andirons in the fieldstone fireplace, and a thick oak mantel.

Peter's wheelchair rests at the dining-room end of the living room, plugged into the wall, recharging, sucking up electricity and giving off an electronic snore. The needle in the window of the charger box, which rests nearby on the floor, has fallen nearly all the way back to "full" position, which means it must be about 3:30 A.M. Knowing what time it is makes insomnia worse, and insomniacs know lots of ways to tell the time.

I move among the furniture, looking for a place, trailing my fingers along the backs of chairs, testing the seats with the flat of my hand. Was Goldilocks an insomniac?

Pausing at the plump wine velvet sofa, I contemplate pulling a fast one. I'll just lie down for a moment and not even think of sleeping, not even try to sleep. I stretch out prone, cross my bare feet at the ankles, place my hands behind my head and slam my eyes shut.

It doesn't work. No sooner do I shut my eyes than there is a fluttering of evil portent in my chest. The lid of a heavy iron box groans open, releasing the hideous beasties of my woe and fury. I am possessed by the forces of my darkest night. They fly at my face, diving at my eyes, catching in my hair, biting, stinging, sucking, poisoning my soul with dread and despair. They test my sanity the way the tongue probes the tooth, to find the fault where the nerve screams and exaggerates it cruelly to the brain.

"Help!" I yell out loud. "I'm cracking up," I say more softly. The moment I hear my words I know them to be true. Here, in the middle of the night, when the rest of the house is sleeping, is when I can hear myself think. I sit up, bring my knees up under my chin, wrap my arms around my legs and stare into the fireplace.

Something's got to give. I just can't do it all. It would be easier if I were willing to have live-in help, but I'm not. I've tried six different housekeepers so far, and they've either quit or been fired or run away. There have been two runaways so far. That's how much they like me, too. It just doesn't work out. I don't let it work out.

I let them clean and shop for groceries and do the wash, but I won't let them take care of Peter—not really. I'm always listening in and intervening when I hear their tempers flare because, after having responded cheerfully through almost five minutes of regrets for painstaking adjustments to Pete's sleeping position ("Fix my ear on the pillow, it's folded under"; "Tuck my right hand more under the pillow"), they find that he *does* have to pee, after all, and they'll have to start all over again.

"Please don't be angry, please, I'm sorry, please," Pete begs after them. The worst thing for Pete is if you're angry with him because it's then that he fears you may desert him, leaving him alone to experience his own helplessness.

I suppose I could try once more. I could put an ad in the paper under "Help Wanted," or maybe just under *"Help!"* I would write the job description very carefully so as to weed out in advance anyone who wasn't right for the job.

Live-in person to help care for ten-year-old boy, wheelchair-bound with muscular dystrophy. Must be loving and cheerful. Must piss child and turn him during the night. Must take the trouble to prop a pillow under his right elbow so that he can hold his penis himself, even though that takes more time. Must cut his food and swoop it through the air like a roller coaster into his mouth, sometimes swerving off at the last minute to fly it into her own mouth instead, to give him something funny to complain about. Must open his bureau drawers each morning and hold up his shirts and trousers, one by one, until he chooses what he wants to wear. (He is getting to that age when he cares about how he looks, especially at school.) Must brush his teeth and not mind if he bites down on a finger. He only does that to show himself, and you, how strong the muscles of his jaws still are, even though the rest of him is wasting. Must, after school, when he tires of entertaining himself by drawing or listening to records, be willing to tell him stories, sing old camp songs, dance around the living room like a klutzy Makarova to Chopin polonaises, or shave his face with aerosol cream and Daddy's empty razor. And if all fails, as sometimes happens, and you sense that the shadow has fallen across his soul, and you know that even you cannot make the sun shine, must hold him in your arms and tell him that you love him, and lift his arms and fold them around your neck so that he can tell you that he loves you too. Best salary for right person.

Of course I've rigged the ad so there can't be any takers, so there isn't any "right" person but me. But there isn't. With all the arrogance of love, I believe that. Nobody else is good enough. Even I'm not good enough.

It's not that I'm determined to be a martyr. It's not that I don't struggle to free myself from my fate at the same time as I embrace it, that I don't sometimes wish Peter dead while I pump life into him, that I don't dream of leaving him while I dig myself in deeper. Even Peter walks in his dreams.

I unclasp my arms from around my legs, lift my head and notice that tears have dampened my nightgown in two round spots where it is stretched taut over my knees. I must have been crying! I really *am* going crazy.

I run from the living room into the front hall, stare into the mirror that hangs on the wall over the lowboy and see a stranger, the same person who stares back at me when I catch her walking by, reflected in a storefront window.

I lean closer toward the mirror. The same red hair. The same dark-brown eyes. She even has freckles, the same kind I've had since I was a kid, not the big splotchy all-year-round kind that go with red hair and pale-green eyes, but the smaller, sprinkles-over-the-bridge-of-the-nose kind that surfaced every summer when I went to camp. She must be me. She even looks as if she's been crying. I reach forward to touch my cheek. The tips of my fingers flatten cold against the mirror's chill surface.

I shiver behind the cold glass screen of the fluoroscope, dressed only in white cotton underpants. My jaw chatters and clatters comically against the machine's chrome frame. I press my chin down hard and clench my teeth to stop the trembling. This is my favorite part of my annual camp physical.

The worst part is when I first come in and have to put the peanut-butter jar containing this morning's urine on Dr. Silverglide's examining table. Then comes the tetanus shot, which will "hardly hurt at all, no worse than a mosquito bite," Mother likes to say. After that, Dr. Silverglide sticks a tongue depressor down my throat until I gag and my face flushes red and hot, and then finally I get to go behind the fluoroscope.

Mother and Dr. Silverglide walk toward me, smiling. He flicks the toggle switch to "on." I am exposed. My insides float on the screen. It is as if I have performed an internal surface dive, my torso following the lunge and scoop of my arms as I cut deep down through the glassy surface and into my shadowy green sea. I see my primordial ferny ocean reflected in a mirror that Dr. Silverglide has installed for "curious children."

I am inside out. There are my ribs. I remember them from last year's camp physical. They are reaching out from the dimly lit depths of me, like the hull of a sunken treasure ship. My spine lurks in the background, mottled and mossy. My hipbones look just like the ones on the paper skeleton that lies in the attic, his jangly joints folded at the grommets, until it's time to hang him on the front door for Halloween.

Was that the day that Pete was born and died? While I stared with wonder and pride, seeing the unseeable me, did that fluoroscope sear the ovum that fifteen years later would be my son? Worse than swift and terrible justice, this punishment would hide inside me like the bullet in the chamber of a gun loaded for Russian roulette. I would pay dearly for this glimpse of the unknowable. My own body would betray me.

Larry likes to cite the doctrine of "last clear chance" to me as exemplary of how exacting and demanding on the individual the law can sometimes be. A driver may be held to be at least partially responsible for an accident, even though it is the other car that has careened out of control, swerved into the oncoming lane and collided head-on with the innocent driver. He is at least partially responsible if it can be demonstrated that he had a last clear chance to avoid the accident.

"You mean," says Adam, "if Pete trips over the leg of a chair, bumps into me, and makes me spill my milk, it could be my fault if I saw him trip and could have moved out of the way?"

"Exactly," says Larry, laying down his fork and shooting me a side glance. I shoot back my fruit-of-the-womb look.

We are two young parents suitable for framing, and here is our first-born, barely four, so smart it would be scary if he weren't so reassuringly normal. Larry is only three years out of law school, and already there are rumors about making him a partner. Home is a small Cape Cod house in a development in Fairfield called Lake Hills where all the young professional couples start out—a cheap property but a good place to begin, like landing on Marvin Gardens after the first roll. A few monopolies and some mortgages later, we expect to land on Westport.

But I worry about Peter. At his checkups in Dr. Braverman's office, he persistently registers "average" and sometimes even "low average" on Dr. Spock's fervently nonjudgmental timetables. He sat up at eight months, took his first steps unassisted at seventeen months, and said his first word at fifteen months.

Adam walked at nine months and said "hot" when he was six months old. Nobody believes me when I tell them, but it's true.

I know it's not fair to compare, but I do. I know it's not right to push, but I can't seem to help it. "How old are you, Petie? Come on, darling, I'll give you a clue." I hold up two fingers. "How many fingers?" Pete just smiles.

He is like a stranger, a shy and serene presence at a boisterous family gathering. He sits quietly at the dinner table, dunking Oreos into his milk while Larry and Adam and I jabber away. I worry that he is not smart.

Each of us sits at one of the four sides of our square mahogany dining-room table. This is the time that Daddy talks to me and my older sister, Carol. In the morning, in the breakfast room, he makes nasal sounds of recognition over the ragged edge of the New York Times, *but it is not until dinnertime that Carol and I actually have an audience. Tonight, between the vichyssoise and the main course, we are going to play my favorite game. It is called "Who will be the apple of Daddy's eye?"*

Daddy leans back in his Chippendale chair, rubs his Phi Beta Kappa key between thumb and index finger and states this evening's problem: "A new client came in to see me yesterday. The evening before his warehouse had burned to the ground, and he wanted me to handle the legal aspects of the matter. Now," says Daddy as the Chippendale lands abruptly on all fours, "which of you girls can tell me what is the very first question to which I need to know the answer before any intelligent analysis of the problem is possible?"

Carol begins to gnaw on her index finger. "You asked him if he had insurance," I answer in an excited, ardent little rush of words, anticipating my reward.

Wrong. Oh my God, I am wrong.

Daddy commences rocking again. All is not lost. He smiles encouragingly at me and pulls on the long hairs in his right eyebrow. I am to be allowed more chances.

"What is the value of the destroyed merchandise?"

Daddy rocks harder and pulls faster.

"Was anybody hurt in the fire?"

The Chippendale ball-and-claw feet are fairly galloping in place on the rug. Impatient, unable to contain himself another moment, Daddy declares, "I asked him whether or not the fire was accidental."

Daddy is in charge of brains. Mother is in charge of social welfare. Both Carol and I can play "Malagueña" for the company before going up to bed, shake hands firmly while looking directly into the other person's eyes, and cross a room with a book on our heads. We are nearly ready.

The subject of tonight's lesson is Forks on the Left, or How to Use a Place Setting. Mother sits up straight in her chair, silent and smiling, until she has our attention. Then she informs us by a tiny dip of her head that she will be teaching by pantomime this evening.

She picks up the salad fork gingerly by its throat, holds it aloft for a studious moment and then lowers it slowly to its place on the table. She does the same for the dinner fork and the dessert fork.

During Mother's lesson I sneak looks at Daddy to see if he has on his cracked-egg look, the face he makes in the morning when he taps open his egg with his knife and finds the white too runny. I can tell that Mother is not the apple of Daddy's eye.

We are the Cohen girls. We are being groomed to marry Warburgs or Rothschilds. "It's just as easy," Mother likes to say, smiling shyly, "to love a rich man as a poor man." She also likes to stress its correlative. "Jews make better husbands."

She has done well. We, her daughters, must do better.

* * *

"Excuse me!" My efforts to shout in a whisper turn every head in the reading room of Goldfarb Library. *"Would anyone here be willing to lend me a car?"* I'm late for a doctor's appointment in Belmont, and mine is stuck in the Harriet and Sidney Rabinowitz Memorial snowdrift in front of Shapiro Hall.

I have promised my father that I will see a psychoanalyst in exchange for being allowed to leave Bryn Mawr and transfer to Brandeis, a move which, to my father's way of thinking, is both reprehensible and pathological, like preferring Tchaikovsky to Mozart.

A bunch of keys jangle and skid down the library table toward me. *"It's the green Buick Dynaflo with the kitchen chair"*—he curls his upper lip over his teeth as if we were conspiring to swipe the Maltese Falcon—*"in front of Slosberg Auditorium."*

I nudge the keys lazily across the last few inches of table and give a tiny salute indicating gratitude and just a hint of tragic wistfulness left over from the last scene of Casablanca. He nudges up the collar on his imaginary trench coat, flicks away a cigarette and, I swear, disappears into the mist. At least I do not see him again for two weeks. And for two weeks I conduct surprise inspections of the reading room, searching for this person who, I've learned, is named Lawrence Paul Weisman.

If he doesn't yet know that he is in love with me, doesn't he even want his car keys back? How can anyone be so offhanded about me, so careless about a car? I learn that he was one of only four Jews on the Brandeis football team, that every morning for two years he strapped tfillin on his arms and one for frontlets between his eyes and then went to Shapiro Athletic Field and ran, headfirst, into the stomachs of two-hundred-pound imported Polish ringers. He majors in comparative literature, lives off campus in a house with five other roommates, one of whom keeps kosher, one of whom crochets, one of whom smoked pot with Norman Mailer, and one who has just gotten a tattoo, which he wrote home about in a letter to his mother, who, in turn, wrote back saying she hoped he was satisfied now that he had broken her heart because he could not be buried in a Jewish cemetery.

Larry Weisman is just what I have been looking for. A bad Jewish boy.

Our wedding is like an album. I seem to have learned the bride's part in some other life. See? I am lifting my Alençon-lace skirts to reveal a satin garter. There is a naughty, come-hither look in my eye.

Here I am feeding a piece of cake to Larry. He is backing off. People around us are laughing. Fun is being had. Larry woke up this morning covered with hives.

In this one I am showing off my engagement ring to Larry's father, my left hand assuming the time-honored, contorted gesture used exclusively by brides and fags. "At least he had the good sense not to bring Barbara," my brain registers snidely, recalling one of the early skirmishes in this doomed but earnest effort to "give Mary-Lou and Larry a lovely wedding" in spite of the fact that everyone else is having a divorce. They are all going to be nice to one another. They have promised.

Take a close look at this picture of Mother standing alone and looking intentionally brave, a face I am used to seeing her assume for public functions and other social martyrdoms when she knows that he is also going to be present. She is disappointed because her daughter, a Cohen girl, is marrying someone who has no money, comes from a broken home and did not go to Harvard.

And here's a candid shot of me in the receiving line. My mother is shaking hands on one side of me. My mother-in-law with her new husband, Eddie, stands on the other. I have already discarded my short net veil and lace-embroidered crown and have retreated behind a Groucho Marx nose-and-eyeglasses disguise. A joke present from a girl friend.

It's the only way I figure I can get through this. We must have been crazy. Whatever made us think that the lofty magic of our love would work like alchemy, transmuting baser mettles into gold.

"Deep pink on the mother of the groom is very inappropriate." Mother turns her head away from the receiving line for a moment to whisper in my ear. Mother is muted in pale aqua.

"Don't let her upset you, darling," Larry's mother is whispering in my other ear.

That's why in this picture I am smiling an ironic smile. I have just figured something out. I am marrying above my station.

Now, this one is a standard shot. Here he *is, leading me down the aisle. My first love. Daddy plays his part shyly, uncomfortably, touchingly. He holds one long white hand lightly at his side, his elbow bent, to receive mine.*

Nobody here can suspect how heady and perilous it is to adore this gentle man, least of all Daddy. Nobody but Daddy's girls can know the archetypal tyranny of his displeasure, as searing as thunderbolts hurled by Zeus. He is going to give me away. He kisses my cheek.

So what's a wedding without music? Surprise! A departure from tradition. An example of that special Cohen touch. See over there behind the cake. It's a string quartet. They are playing Mozart. But it is not until Larry's Aunt Fanny applauds the first movement and politely requests a hora *that I think we would have been more realistic to elope.*

"Well," says Adam, setting down his milk glass on the dinner table, "I don't think the law of last clear chance is fair. I think that when Pete trips and falls and makes me spill my milk, it would be all Pete's fault. I think that Pete is a doo-doo."

Adam and Peter look solemn for a moment, and then they giggle their milk up their noses and run sputtering and galloping around the kitchen, Denton toes flapping.

"Okay, youze guys." I get up from the table and start to clear the dishes. "Intobedyougo. And," I add, sticking out my lower lip as far as I can, "as the Ubangi mother said to her children, 'Don't give me any of your lip.' Daddy'll tuck you in."

"Do it again, Daddy, do it again!" Pete chortles as Larry bends over him, presses his face into Pete's milk-sticky belly and blows, making unpredictable, staccato noises. "Blibble my tummy one more time."

Pete lies on his back in bed and grins his sneaky grin. Tiny white teeth glisten with saliva, sparkling and pure as water from a wilderness stream splashing over sunlit mica pebbles.

Saliva. Mouth water, as Pete calls it. See what innocence and beauty can do for spit.

The corners of his wide grin stretch his pouty cheeks out and upward, until the sprinkling of Huck Finn freckles forms crescents that almost eclipse his round, hazel eyes. Laughter wrinkles his tiny, pointed nose into a V. Suddenly, soulful chipmunk face turns into beamy pumpkin puss. He wiggles his legs with excess, daffy delight. His rubber pants crinkle and crunch.

And Larry and I laugh at the best joke of all—that we, the two of us, should have created this miracle, this perfection, this child.

Larry smiles up shyly at me and goes down once more, waggling his head faster and faster as the quacks and gurgles escape into thin air.

"You know what they sound like, Daddy?" Pete giggles wickedly.

"I can't imagine," Larry leers. "Come on, Pockie, it's after your bedtime."

"Farts," says Peter. "They sound like farts. Daddy?"

"What, Pete?"

"Daddy, what's a last clear chance?"

"It's all you've got left before I come in here and blibble you and your tummy all the way to Kingdom Come."

"Dr. Braverman will be with you shortly, Mrs. Weisman," says the nurse. "He's just finishing up a camp physical."

I slide Pete off my hip and settle him on a tiny wicker chair in front of the educationally suitable challenge of a brightly painted wooden Fisher-Price mailbox, but not before the sweet stench of bowel movement mixed with Baby Magic invades my lungs.

"Oh, Pete," I chide softly, pleadingly. "I just asked you before we left home. Why don't you make your doo-doos in the toilet? You're almost two and a half years old; you're a big boy now. Don't you want to poop in the toilet like Adam and Mommy and Daddy?"

"No," says Pete, holding a square peg in his pudgy grasp and rotating it with great determination at the mouth of a round hole.

"Why not?" I ask. I never thought to ask why not before.

"Because I like it," he comments from his trance of concentration, still turning the peg patiently around and around. "It feels warm, and soft, and squishy."

"Well," I admit with a weak smile, prying the square peg from his clutch and replacing it with the round one, "that's an answer at least." The peg drops into the mailbox with a clunk.

Like Gulliver in Lilliput, I perch on a chair next to Pete, my knees at my chin, and stare at the seam in the wallpaper where Christopher Robin's foot has been lopped off in midstride. Nearby, Edward Bear buries his snoot in a jar labeled "Hunny," and Tigger leaps for joy. In the corner, fat goldfish flirt and unfurl their fins in a rectangular glass world of bubbles and blue gravel. Hanging in front of the large, sunny window in a colorfully beaded macramé sling, a spider plant throws out little tufted explosions of green growth.

There's probably nothing wrong with him, I think, my eyes wandering back to Christopher Robin's neatly severed ankle. It's probably just my imagination. I'm a worrier. This is a happy place, where mothers complain of sneezles and wheezles and what is the matter with Mary Jane, and a lump is a mump, not a tumor. And the reason that Pete waddles when he walks, for Chrissakes, is because he always has a load in his pants! I feel so foolish that I consider leaving.

The phone buzzes behind the reception counter and the nurse picks up. "Dr. Braverman will see you now," she says and holds open the door to Dr. Braverman's office.

"Hi, pal," says Dr. Braverman, taking Pete from my arms and setting him down on the scale.

Dr. Braverman is one of the new breed of young, designer

physicians, eschewing the starched white jacket or business suit for faded but ironed jeans, a velour shirt, gold chain and top-siders. He wears a Mickey Mouse watch and rewards each tearless injection or unprotested probe of the tongue depressor with a balloon, which he blows up with a foot pump.

"Let's see how big you've gotten since last time." He fiddles with the sliding arrow until the weights balance and the arrow indicates thirty-three pounds. "You really like to pack it away, pal, don't you?" Pete just smiles.

"You can deduct about five pounds for the load in his pants," I demur.

Dr. Braverman walks behind his desk to record the weight on Pete's chart. "What brings you here today, Mary-Lou?" He gestures toward a facing chair, upholstered in red patent leather. "Sit down, sit down, please."

"Actually, I feel kind of silly, now that I'm here. I don't think anything's wrong, really, but I've noticed lately that Pete seems to be a little unsteady on his feet. He bumps into things. Maybe there's something wrong with his legs, or maybe his eyes, or maybe he's just a klutz."

"C'mere, Pete," says Dr. Braverman, reaching out his arms. "C'mon over here and let me take a good look at you. You're almost as big as your brother, aren't you?"

Pete walks steadily toward Dr. Braverman, who holds up two fingers. "How many fingers?"

Pete just smiles.

"One or two?"

"Two."

"Right-o," beams Dr. Braverman. "That's as old as you are, isn't it?"

"I'm almost two and a half," Pete announces, "and I still poop in my pants."

"That's what I like, a kid with a mind of his own." Braverman chuckles, looking into Pete's eyes with a flashlight, moving the light up and down, right and left. "They look okay to me," he says, turning off the light. "Funny, I thought maybe you were right about his eyes. They had a strange, sort of lazy look from across the room, but they look fine. I don't detect any weakness in the muscles." He bends down to push Pete's trouser legs. He runs his hands slowly up and down each leg, and as his hand passes over Peter's calf, I think I see his smile fade.

"What about his legs?"

"They look pretty good to me too, but just to be on the safe side, why don't you take him to see Bruce Devlin—he's a good orthopedic man—and for good measure, we'll have Barry Blakely take a more comprehensive look at his eyes. We don't want any anxious mothers in Westport."

"Bloon," says Pete, sensing that the visit is over.

"What's your favorite color?" Dr. Braverman asks, reaching into his balloon drawer.

"Puce."

"Adam put him up to that," I explain, laughing. "Make it red."

"I'll let you know what the doctors have to say, if anything," says Braverman, ushering us out the door.

A house call these days is as rare as a telegram from the White House. It can mean your son is dying.

"Muscular," says Dr. Braverman. "I assume that part is clear enough. Self-explanatory, actually. Now dystrophy. Dystrophy refers to the atrophying of the muscles in a distended position." Removing his fingertips from his shoulders like a cheerleader, he extends his forearms until they are perfectly straight, parallel to the floor.

For one moment he hangs like a charade in the middle of our living room. It must be my turn to guess.

"Is muscular dystrophy a terminal disease?" I ask, trying to demonstrate simultaneously that I am a good learner and that I can be trusted to handle with professional tact and detachment what must be a very uncomfortable situation. I can see that Dr. Braverman already looks a lot more at ease than when I opened the front door and saw him standing there, hands plunged into the pockets of his jean jacket.

"Not exactly," he answers. "One doesn't die from muscular dystrophy. One dies from pneumonia. The pneumonia results from the eventual atrophying of the muscles of the lungs, rendering them unable to expel mucus effectively." Charming! I respect a person who has a good command of the nuances of the English language. There is this disease called muscular dystrophy (MD for short)—perhaps you've seen the Jerry Lewis telethon or noticed the disease on a canister at your cleaners?—and this disease is born with the baby, and it grows with the baby. As the baby's muscles develop, the disease eats those muscles, turning them into fat. To grow is to die. But wait! That's not quite right. Muscular dystrophy, MD for short, doesn't exactly kill you. It only makes you gradually and completely limp, so limp that you cannot hold a pencil. So limp that you cannot wave goodbye. So limp outside and in that I can hardly hear you sneeze. So limp that one day you will catch a cold, the kind of cold that for a normal kid means wiping his nose on a sleeve, and it will kill you by turning into pneumonia, and it will be the pneumonia, not the MD, that will actually do the killing. And your death will be as slow as your lifetime of dying. You will first strain slightly for breath and then there will be panic whirling in your eyes, and then you will gasp and you will say with your dying breath, "Help me, Mommy, I can't breathe," but I won't be able to help you and you will die.

But I don't say any of these things out loud, or even to myself. We have agreed to pretend that nothing is happening, and a deal is a deal. Instead I ask, "At about what age does the average person afflicted with MD die?" I congratulate myself on the clarity and objectivity of the question.

"That," says Dr. Braverman, "is not easy to answer. Prior to the discovery of penicillin," he says soberly, as if reciting the Preamble to the Constitution, "children with muscular dystrophy—Duchenne type, which I suspect Peter has—seldom lived beyond their early teens. Now, however, they can live considerably longer."

Considerably longer. Am I hearing good news? Considerably longer enough to ride a ten-speed, fall in love, get married, have children, see them grow? Considerably longer enough to have lived a normal lifetime in, say, medieval times, when people didn't normally live beyond forty years anyway? Considerably longer enough for me to think of it that way?

I clear my throat. "Could you be just a little more specific as to how long 'considerably longer' is, for instance, in years?"

I can see that he doesn't like that question. I should not have tried to put him on the spot. How are we all going to be able to pretend that nothing is happening if we have to answer specific questions like that? But it's too late. The question has been asked, so it must be answered. "You must realize, of course, that it is impossible for me to be specific. Each case is individual. He might live into his third decade."

I try to understand "third decade" but I am notoriously bad with numbers. Sometimes I can't remember if the eighteenth century is the seventeen-hundreds or the nineteen-hundreds. How many candles on a birthday cake is "third decade"? But my mind jams. Third decade. Considerably longer. Miracle drug. Not exactly terminal.

Are there any more questions? Yes, if you don't mind terribly much, if you're not already too disgusted with me. Just give me another chance. You'll see, I can do better.

"Is the brain in any way affected by muscular dystrophy?"

"No." He smiles reassuringly, happy to be the harbinger of such good news. "Every part of the body is affected, I believe, except the head."

"What about bowel and bladder control?" I ask, my questions trying to punch this yeasty tragedy down to a manageable size. Will he always be in diapers? Will he be able to bite his food? And isn't the heart a muscle like the lungs? And if the heart is muscle like the lungs, don't they all just go limp and couldn't his heart just get too limp to beat and couldn't that happen before his lungs get too limp to breathe and wouldn't that be a much less awful way to die than sucking for faint strands of air?

"I really don't know if there is any involvement of the bowel and bladder at any stage of the disease," says Dr. Braverman, reaching the end of his professional rope and his tolerance for this scene simultaneously. "Some of your more specific questions would be better answered by Dr. Tierney in New York, who is a specialist in this field. It would also be wise to have him confirm my diagnosis. I will call him in the morning and make an appointment for you. My nurse will be in touch . . . I think that I have stayed long enough. I'll leave you now," he says, backing toward the door, tucking his hands back into his pockets.

"I'm sorry," I hear him say as I quietly press the door closed behind him.

"Thank you so much for coming," I reply, not yet aware that this was our first condolence call.

This is a test, an easy test, a baby test. It is so easy you cannot study for it. If you get it right, you fail. If you flunk, you pass.

"Now, Peter, I'm going to sit you on the floor like so, and when I say, 'Ready, get set, go,' I want you to stand up as quickly as you can. Okay?" says Dr. Tierney, placing Pete plunk in the middle of his examining room floor.

"Okay," says Peter.

"Ready, get set . . . go!" shouts Dr. Tierney gaily. Pete, still seated, smiles his readiness to cooperate, rotates deliberately to his right, places both palms flat on the floor, pushes against the floor until his legs straighten and his bottom is high in the air, slow motion, like an instant replay. I suppress an urge to hiss in his ear, "For Chrissakes, Petie, get up faster. You can do better than that." Then, releasing one hand at a time from the floor, he quickly transfers them to his own knees where he gives one more almost imperceptible push, and he is standing.

"Very good," says Dr. Tierney, "that's very good. You are a very good boy." But I can tell he has gotten it right, right for MD.

"Now," says Dr. Tierney, "let's see if you can whistle."

Pete puckers up and whistles.

"Terrific," cheers Dr. Tierney. Larry and I exchange nervous smiles. Being able to whistle must be a good sign, a terrific sign. Hooray! Pete has flunked.

"Ooop-la!" strains Dr. Tierney as he hoists Pete onto the examining table. "Now," says the doctor, reaching into the pocket of his lab coat, "let's see what I've got for you in here."

Peter, lollypop-expectant and confused, reaches for the little red rubber hammer and lifts it to his mouth.

"No, silly," say I, joining in on the fun, "it's a hammer. Bang! Bang! A hammer, a hammer, bang, bang, a hammer," and I do not realize until Larry reaches over and puts his hand on my knee that I can hardly stop talking.

Dr. Tierney bangs the hammer first on the palm of his own hand, then on Peter's; next on his own knee, and then on Peter's.

"It dozints hurts," says Pete reassuringly.

I watch Dr. Tierney crouched near Peter's knee, tapping and pausing, tapping and pausing, like a prisoner signaling a cellmate in code through concrete. Pausing, ear pressed, head cocked, Dr. Tierney smiles blindly into the air, squinting, expectant, not breathing, waiting after each tap for an answer, a "Who's there?," a sign of life.

Finally he slips the hammer back into his pocket, casually, even cavalierly, as if trying to make the gesture of giving up look as much as possible like merely stopping. Peter has flunked the reflex test.

"Sometimes doctors can't find my reflexes either, and I'm still here," says Larry loyally, foolishly.

Dr. Tierney picks Peter up in his arms and turns to take a chair behind his desk. He is about to tell us the score.

Is this the end of the test? Aren't there any more questions, any multiple choices, any essay questions? (I always do well on the essay questions.) Are there going to be any extra credit questions? Is this just a true or false test? Will there be a make-up test? Oh please don't stop asking questions, please play more games, play more games, please, I want to cry out. Make Peter whistle again. Come on, Peter, whistle for Dr. Tierney. He's a terrific whistler, Dr. Tierney, perhaps you didn't notice. But my own desperation silences me.

Dr. Tierney leans back in his leather chair until the springs scream. "A diagnosis of muscular dystrophy at age two and a half is astute, extremely astute. I'm sorry to say, Dr. Braverman's diagnosis is correct," he tells me without wincing as Peter, nestled comfortably on his lap, bangs intently on his kneecaps with a hammer.

My eyes lock onto Dr. Tierney's face, searching, casting, rummaging, begging for something more, something else, something especially for me, saved for last, best for last, that will mean this isn't really happening. Dr. Tierney meets my gaze directly for a moment and then blinks and flinches. "Down you go," says Dr. Tierney.

Peter slides, belly down, from Dr. Tierney's lap, his toes wiggling to seek the floor.

"Fanks," says Pete, handing the hammer back to Dr. Tierney. "Fanks a lot." And Pete runs laboriously toward me, flinging himself forward intently with each step, his silky auburn hair moving like liquid under the fluorescent hospital lights.

As he pulls himself onto my lap I feel my gorge rise. He leans against my chest. I compensate by supporting the soles of his feet in the palms of my hands. I am covered with sweat. I swallow repeatedly behind my firm smile. Saliva surges and aches in my jaws. Peter is making me sick. I cannot stand to feel him. I cannot stand to touch him.

"Go to Daddy, Pete," I say, sliding him down my legs. "Go to Daddy."

Larry reaches his arms out like a sleepwalker. His features seem disordered, angry and bewildered, as if he has just inadvertently walked into cobwebs.

I look to Dr. Tierney, my expression so cordial it is almost brazen, my lips inviting, even daring him to say more, to go on, my eyes perfectly defying and betraying my gut, encouraging him to believe that I am coping very well.

"Now," says Dr. Tierney, taking me at my unspoken word, "although I am one hundred percent sure of the diagnosis, I would like to arrange for some further, more definitive tests: a creatine phosphokinase, or CPK, test, a muscle biopsy and an electromyogram. Positive responses to these tests will mean we can have absolute confidence in the diagnosis."

"What is creatine phosphokinase?" I ask automatically, barely noticing that I do not care in the least how he answers this question. The point, as in some detective story, is to keep him talking while I figure out how to get us out of here.

"CPK is an enzyme confined almost exclusively to muscle. Therefore, if we find unusually elevated amounts of this creatine phosphokinase in the blood serum, we can assume leakage from the muscle tissue."

My mind is wandering. My eyes scan his office, looking for clues about who he is, where I am, and how to be. The requisite photo of wife and children, shoulder overlapping shoulder, posed on the bias in descending order, is missing. The sounds of traffic on 168th Street are random, remote and unfamiliar. There are no books on his desk. There is no philodendron for his secretary to water. The telephone does not ring. I am losing my bearings.

I look to Larry. His face has changed utterly. The fragments have reorganized. He sits alert and obedient in his chair, as if by paying careful attention to what Dr. Tierney is telling him about the disease, he can learn how to cure it. Pete sits at Larry's feet, untying his shoelaces.

I ask some more questions, just to keep myself from disappearing. "What about the muscle biopsy? What is involved? Does he have to go to the hospital? How long will he be in the hospital? Can I stay with him if he has to stay overnight?" I pepper Dr. Tierney with inquisitorial shrapnel, calculated to demonstrate deep maternal love and concern, when what I am actually feeling is a bewildering sense of detachment, panic and nausea.

"He'll have to be an inpatient, but just for three or four days, just long enough to complete the requisite tests," says Dr. Tierney, adding reassuringly, "He'll be in the pediatric ward, so he'll have plenty of company. We find that other children are the best hospital company for children, even better than their mothers."

I am relieved to hear this, although I affect a look of thoughtfulness, tempered with reticence which I demonstrate by chewing a bit on my lower lip. I do not want to stay in the hospital with Peter. I do not want to be anywhere with Peter. I cannot stomach my own child.

"Well," I say, "if you're sure that your experience bears out the contention that Pete will be better off in the children's ward . . ."

"I'm absolutely sure," says Dr. Tierney.

"Of course I can visit him, can't I?"

"Of course," he says. "Just about any time you want to. The hospital policy is very liberal about visiting hours, especially when children are involved."

"That's good," I say, smiling as if mollified.

"It might also be wise if you underwent some tests yourself," says Dr. Tierney, shifting in his chair, recrossing his legs, and making the fingers of his right and left hands perform little push-ups against one another. "I will refer you to a geneticist, Dr. Kittenplan at Mount Sinai, if you like. Muscular dystrophy is a recessive, sex-linked disease, transmitted through the female but affecting predominantly male offspring. Up to fifty percent of male children may develop the disease, while fifty percent of female children, like yourself, may be carriers."

As he speaks a large pigeon flies out of his mouth, the kind of pigeon that often sits on top of one of the marble lions' heads in front of the New York Public Library, main branch, the kind of pigeon I always fear will be startled by my footfall and fly, with a wild rush of beating wings and pecking beak, into my face. But all at once this pigeon melts and smooths into a dove, the dove that winged its way toward Noah. Warm and white, it descends gently, landing on my lap. There is a tiny roll of paper attached to its thin pink leg, tinier even than the marvelously minute copy of the Ten Commandments that I once extracted with my mother's tweezers from the mezuzah alongside our front door.

I remove the message from its leg. It reads: "Not guilty."

"I don't know of anyone in our family who had muscular dystrophy," I say, hastily trying to put together in my mind a genealogy of Perelmutter family diseases. I never really knew Baba, Great Grandma Perelmutter, but I know she died of one of the whispered words, cancer. Her daughter Bessie, my Grandma Perelmutter, is the one who emigrated from Russia to New Haven by way of Winnipeg.

"What about your maternal grandmother?" says Dr. Tierney.

"All of her children were healthy." I smile, remembering Grandma Perelmutter.

I see her, pacing back and forth across the kitchen floor, glass in hand, taking dainty sips of her special water from Saratoga. We both wait patiently for that lusty, rambunctious burp, rising from her depths, that heralds Grandma's essential physical well-being. When it comes, we both laugh.

"Wonderful," she pronounces, laying a heavy but graceful hand on her huge bosom, like a diva who has just completed an aria. "You should always take care of your health. Health and *mazel*. Do you know what *mazel* means, darling?" she asks me for the millionth time. "Luck!" she answers for me. "Good health and good luck. That is all you need."

"My maternal grandparents were Russian immigrants," I tell Dr. Tierney. "I suppose my grandmother's mother, the one who died of cancer, might have had children we don't know about, perhaps even a male child, who did not survive early childhood, or maybe even died at birth, who might have had MD." I say this, but I don't believe it. I do not believe that there could be something so awful, so deadly, so secret, locked in my genes.

"Right," says Dr. Tierney. "That's all the more reason why you should undergo some tests, to determine whether or not you are a carrier. But first, let's test out this little fellow," he chucks Pete under the chin, venturing into pediatric jocularity, a sign I recognize as meaning "Your time is up."

I am not ready to go. I cannot be dismissed from this place into my life. I cannot imagine my life.

"Is there anything to do?" I ask. "Any treatment at all?"

"Not really," he says, "not now. In a few years, when he is having difficulty walking, we can discuss the advisability of a heel-cord operation. You see, the Achilles tendon becomes foreshortened, causing the child to walk on his toes. At that time we can operate, and cut the Achilles tendon. Then, with the use of braces, we are able to keep these children walking and put off the necessity of a wheelchair for a year or two. But that's something we don't have to worry about right now," he says, ushering us to the door. I get it. Act as if nothing is happening.

That night we lie together, side by side, not touching, strangers, estranged, no longer recognizing ourselves, no longer recognizing each other, no longer young. Uncomforting, uncomfortable, I pretend to be asleep.

I hear a tiny voice, a silly little blubbering noise, the boo-hooing of a small, sweet child whose ice cream, a reward perhaps for being good, has just toppled from the cone at a touch of his eager, innocent tongue. It is the despairing, inconsolable noise before the mother says, "Don't cry darling, Mommy will buy you another," and miraculously consoles, leaving the child to deal with those last few uncalled-for gulps and gasps and heaves that have not yet quite understood that "everything is going to be all right" and that "there is nothing to cry about."

Only Larry, the child, that tear-shiny, chapped-cheek child I never met, knows how to cry. It is the man and father Larry who recognizes what the sobbing child inside cannot know; that this is beyond his or any grownup's capacity to make it better. "You know what keeps running through my mind?" he sobs.

"What, darling?"

"That Peter will never know what it's like to make love to a woman."

I turn my head toward his sorrow. I see rationed tears, a judicious few forced out by sheer pressure and without consent, travel down his temples, disappear into thick, curly black hair and meander across his scalp and into the pillow. His sculpted head, its perfectly calculated brow, cheekbone and jaw, as if calibrated according to some classic formula, glows like a medallion, lit by the faint glow of moonlight filtering through the window.

He is holding on to his penis with both hands, pulling it harshly. "Oh my poor baby," he keens, "oh my poor baby."

When at last Larry falls asleep I stare at the ceiling, the sheet folded beneath my chin, my mind cleared of thought, full of emptiness, waiting for sleep to draw its palm over my eyes. All night I try on familiar images of sorrow: a telephone receiver abruptly abandoned, dangling in the air on its spiral cord—thick, raw hands twisting a handkerchief near a mine shaft in West Virginia—the face of Anne Frank—then, a newspaper photograph of a Vietnamese mother holding her dead infant in outstretched arms, as if it were an offering to Reuters.

"Did you sleep well?" I ask Larry solicitously the next

morning, as if I am reading the lines of a middle-aged matron from some theater-of-the-absurd one-act play. And he
answers back, as if he, too, holds the same script, as if we are
both trying out for the same play, walking through the lines.
"Fine."

"What can I make you for breakfast?" I say.

"I don't think I feel like breakfast today," he says courteously.

"What do you feel like!" I scream, throwing away the
script, reaching for his sleeve.

"Like shit," he says, and we lean against each other, my
cheek against his pin-striped shoulder, his cheek against my
bathrobe, our arms hanging at our sides.

"We are going to be all right," says Larry, straightening
up. "We're going to be all right," he repeats. "We'll talk tonight. I've got to run now. I'm on trial."

I recognize the game. I know the rules. Act as if nothing
has happened.

Quietly I open the door to the children's bedroom and
take in the familiar picture, a voyeuristic moment of innocence and beauty before they awaken. Four-year-old Adam
is sleeping in his junior bed, clutching his flannel blanket.
Peter sleeps in his crib, thumb in mouth. I watch him sleep. I
watch as his thumb begins to slide out of his mouth. I see the
muscle in his cheek begin to throb, drawing the thumb back
into position. This tender baby drama of panic and reassurance plays over and over again to its happy conclusion. I
move closer to his crib. I revel in the spill of gleaming auburn hair across his smoky, poreless brow. I examine the
perfection of each eyelash and locate its origin in the crescent
of each lid. I relish the sweet comedy of freckles scattered on
his cheeks and nose, and the segmented roundness of firm,
satiny limbs. They tempt me to believe that all is well, that
nothing, indeed, has happened.

What is wrong with this picture? Just after Follow the
dots, and Find your way out of the maze, and How many
birds can you find in this tree?, there was always a "What is

wrong with this picture?" So where is the gash to match the gash in me? Where are the screams to match the screams in me?

Sometimes it was tricky—a matter of no doorknob on the door, or maybe where the little girl and boy sat coloring there were only three legs on the table, or perhaps just one sock on the little girl, but it was always there and I could always find it. It was never invisible. It was never like this. It was never a worm under the skin.

I turn and hold the knob and pull the door closed silently. I lean against the wall and try to quiet the raucous echoes in my head, the roaring emptiness in my stomach, to impose some order.

It is, I tell myself, only Tuesday. Tuesday, May 2, 1967. It is not all the days of the week, all the years of his life, and everything that is going to happen is not happening all at once. It is merely now, 1967, May 2, Tuesday, 8 A.M. It is time to make coffee.

"Mommy, soakinvet! Mommy, soakinvet!" Peter yells from his crib. I press the slightly parted fingers of my left hand hard against my open, gagging mouth and breathe in and out noisily until the forced breathing overpowers the threat of bile rising in the back of my throat.

I come through his door as a good-morning smile, scoop him up from his crib and press him against my revulsion. The silk of his skin might as well be scales.

"Silly old Pockety-Pock," I say over his shoulder, tears streaming uncried out of my eyes. "Why do you keep on pissing in your diapers?"

"Mommy fik-its," says Pete, comforting both of us.

"You're right, little Fudgetickle Entworth LaRue, poor tired work-her-fingers-to-the-bone Mommy will, faster than you can say 'presto chango,' fik-its."

"Chango-pwesto," says Peter.

He lies, belly up, on his outgrown bathinette, plump, firm arms waving, diaper-parted legs kicking gently, lackadaisically, at the air. I take a deep breath and hold it. Tentatively I press my face against his downy cheek, curl my lips to nibble on his ear lobe, his nipples, touch his bellybutton with my tongue, kiss the insides of his damp thighs.

Suddenly, in a rush, love escapes from my lungs, spills from my body, pouring abundantly over his. More and more gasps forth from me. I am well where, just a moment ago, I was sick. I am astounded with what abandon my body gives up love and breath and still finds more to lavish. It is a miracle. Maybe we *are* going to be all right.

The telephone rings.

"I'll get it!" Adam calls eagerly from downstairs. "Weisman residumps, Adam Weisman speaking . . . Oh, hi, Mangie. Mom's upstairs with Pete. I'll get her . . . It's okay. She's not busy." "Mangie" is what Adam calls my mother.

"I'll diaper you later, Pockie. Mangie's on the phone." I place Peter on the floor. "Tell her to hang on," I call down, checking my face in the mirror. I don't want Adam to know I've been crying. I stare intently into my eyes. The puffiness could as easily be sleepiness as sorrow. "I'll be down in a jiffy."

But I move slowly down the stairs, the damp palm of my hand alternately sticking and then dragging against the varnished wood banister as it follows the rest of me, reluctantly. I am not ready to tell Mother. I am not ready to tell anyone.

What is this flutter of sensation in my chest—almost like panic, but not quite—that makes me want to draw the drapes, lock the door, take the phone off the hook and hide? I am a victim, not a criminal. So why do I feel so ashamed?

"Hi, Mom."

"Aren't you going to ask me how I am?"

"How are you?"

"I've been better. My sinuses are acting up."

"I'm sorry."

"Is something wrong, dear? You sound preoccupied."

"Hang on just a second, Mom." I cover the mouthpiece of

the phone. "Addie, go on upstairs and keep Peter cumps while I'm talking to Mangie, will you?"

"You mean 'Get lost'?"

"I mean 'Get lost' and I love you." I give Adam a potch in the tush and he runs upstairs on all fours.

"Mom? Are you there?" I stall. I don't know how to do this. My life feels like theater. "Perhaps you'd better sit down. I have something to tell you . . ."

"You're not pregnant again, are you, dear?"

"No, Mom."

"That's good. You have your hands full as it is. I'm sitting down, darling. What is it?"

"We took Peter to see a specialist in New York yesterday. We've been concerned because Pete's been walking kind of strangely, you know, clumsily . . . and he examined Peter . . . and he's pretty sure he's got a very serious disease, a terminal disease called muscular dystrophy. It destroys muscle tissue. First he'll be in a wheelchair and then he'll get pneumonia and then he'll die." I wail like a baby. "Oh, Mommy, what am I going to do?"

"Mary-Lou, dear . . . Mary-Lou . . . dear, calm down for a minute."

I muzzle my mouth with my hand, gasping for air between clenched fingers.

"That's better. Now then, dear, what's this doctor's name and hospital affiliation?"

"Tierney, Dr. Amos Tierney. He's in the department of neurology at Columbia Presbyterian."

Mother sends a whoosh of air through her nostrils. Tierney is not a Jewish name. Columbia Presbyterian is not Mount Sinai. "This doctor is not aba-so-lute-ly positive of his diagnosis, is he?"

"He's almost positive. They have to do some tests to be absolutely positive."

"There, you see? You're prematurely upset. You don't even know if Peter has this disease. Doctors can be wrong, you know. Remember the Alexander girl from Hamden?

Four doctors from Yale diagnosed her problem as thyroid, and meanwhile she was eating ice cream directly from the freezer in the basement. Remember, dear, you come from good, healthy stock."

"Maybe not such good, healthy stock, Mom. Muscular dystrophy is a hereditary disease, carried in the mother's genes."

"Nonsense! He couldn't have gotten it from our side. Don't jump to conclusions. Wait until they've done the tests, and even then, get a second opinion. Now pull yourself together, dear."

"Okay, Mom."

"That's my daughter!" Mother brags. "One more thing, dear . . ."

"What?"

"Don't tell anybody about this; at least not yet."

"Why not?"

"There's no need to broadcast it. The less people know about your business, the better."

"Okay, Mom."

"Goodbye, dear."

"Goodbye, Mom."

"And remember, dear. Not a word to anyone."

"Okay, Mom."

"There's a brave girl."

There is a click, punctuated by the nasal hum of the dial tone.

The roar of the Electrolux fills the den. The tank, responding to Mother's sudden tugs at the hose, heels like a beaten dog. She pushes the nozzle of the vacuum cleaner back and forth, back and forth, scrubbing at the medallion on the rug as if it were a stain. She reminds me of a story Grandpa Perelmutter likes to tell me when we're playing gin rummy, of how some Russian Jews escaped across Europe, pumping away at a railroad handcart. Even though Eddie Mae comes in every day, Mother likes to vacuum.

"Mother!" I holler above the noise. My voice seems very loud to me, but it does not reach Mother's ears. She crouches, ramming the nozzle in and out under the love seat.

"Mother!" I yell again, louder. "Muh-uh-uh-ther!" I shout, clenching my fists. I follow the tank following her, my shouts disappearing into the white noise of the vacuum cleaner.

At last, she stomps on the tank button with one foot, like the victor stepping on the vanquished's chest, jerks the plug out of the socket with one deft yank and sends it whiplashing, convulsing, across the floor toward her.

"Did you want something, Mary-Lou?" She looks into my face as if she had just awakened from a dream.

"Nothing," I mutter.

"Now then, what did you want?"

"I wanted you to read to me."

"At ten o'clock in the morning? Why don't you go outside and play?"

"It's raining."

"What about your friend Pam?"

"Her mother says she's still contagious."

"All right," Mother sighs, weaving the cord into figure eights between her elbow and the crotch of her thumb. "Get the book. And hurry up. The Smith Club is coming soon."

Mother sits down. I snuggle up against her purple-and-gray tweed suit. This is the time I love. This is when I am close to her. Sometimes she lets me rub the palm of my hand up and down her silky shin, feeling the prickly stubble of shaved hairs poking through the nylon.

" 'Once there was an Indian named brave Mr. Buckingham. He was called brave Mr. Buckingham because he was very, very, very brave—' " She interrupts her reading for a warning: "Careful not to give me a run, dear."

" 'And no matter how frightfully terrible an accident was that happened to him, brave Mr. Buckingham just smiled a brave smile and he said, "That didn't hurt!" ' " Mother reads with expression. She used to teach elocution to children in her home before she had Carol and me.

" 'One day Mr. Buckingham was playing a blindfold game, and he held his foot up to see if he could guess what it was that made such a *nice tickly feeling like air blowing . . . all of a sudden he felt another feeling, only not tickly, and it was his foot being cut off.' "*

I look at the picture on the right-hand side. Mr. Buckingham is holding his foot up against the rotary blade of a buzz saw.

" 'But brave Mr. Buckingham smiled a brave smile and he said . . .' " Here Mother smiles, inviting me with a solicitous little prod of a nod to recite along with her on the refrain: " 'That didn't hurt.' " Then she reads on.

" 'One day Mr. Buckingham went to the aquarium because he wanted to find if fishes can tell time, and he jumped in with a quite large fish and he asked, "What time does my watch say?" And the fish said, "Dinner time!" and he bit Mr. Buckingham's foot right off and ate it. But brave Mr. Buckingham smiled a brave smile, and he said . . .' " Mother encourages me with a solemn, slight bow of her head to join in, and together we sing-song, " 'That didn't hurt!' "

Page by page, picture by picture, limb by limb, "That didn't hurt" by "That didn't hurt," brave Mr. Buckingham loses his parts. While he is trimming the hollyhocks, the pincers slip and pinch off one of his arms. A kitchen accident burns brave Mr. Buckingham's leg off, right to the top of the thigh. A saw, carelessly thrown from an airplane, saws Mr. Buckingham's hand off. Finally, one day when a handless, footless, armless, legless Mr. Buckingham is taking a sunbath in the middle of the road, a truck comes along and slices his body off.

And after each accident, Mother's voice rises in elocuted horror and surprise, and then our voices join in a crescendo of incredulity and joyous pronunciamento: " 'That didn't hurt!' "

On the last page there's nothing left of brave Mr. Buckingham except a head. Just a head, a neatly severed head, set on a kitchen table. He is wearing a headband with eight jaunty feathers. His lips smile. His eyes twinkle merrily. A little girl stands nearby, spooning large ripe strawberries into his mouth.

" 'And that was the very last terrible accident that brave Mr. Buckingham ever had. After that he lived happily, happily ever after, and whenever he was hungry, his dear little granddaughter would help Mr. Buckingham to eat a big plateful of beautiful red strawberries, because strawberries were brave Mr. Buckingham's favorite thing. And brave Mr. Buckingham was so used to saying, "That didn't hurt,"

that as soon as he had eaten the last beautiful strawberry, he smiled a
very, very brave smile, and he said' "—and here Mother turns the last
page with a slow, parabolic flourish while we both recite the last few
words by heart, straight ahead into the air, " 'That didn't hurt!' " and
she closes the book.

"Where does he swallow to?" I ask.

"What do you mean?"

"I mean, brave Mr. Buckingham doesn't have a stomach to swallow
the strawberries into, and besides that, he doesn't have a place where
he can make—"

"That's quite enough, young lady. That will be quite enough."

"Poo-poo!" I giggle. "He has no place to make—"

Smash! Her palm stings my cheek. My eyes fill. I stare straight
ahead as if nothing has happened. I do not flinch, I do not even blink.
That way, no tears will escape.

"Fuck you!" I sob into the dead receiver and hang it up
resoundingly. I sit down on the kitchen floor, hug myself
around the legs, rest my forehead on my knees and cry until
I'm done. Have mercy on your mother, says my nicest voice.
She's even more scared than you are.

I hear the sound of a toilet flushing and of Peter's singsong
voice crooning, "Bye, bye, doo-doo, bye, bye, doo-doo."

"Peter!" I call out with excitement, getting up off the
floor. "Did you make in the toilet like a big boy?"

"No," Adam's cynical voice answers from the top of the
stairs. "First he pooped on the hall floor like a baby. *Then* he
went into the bathroom and flushed the toilet like a big
boy."

"Mommy fik-its!" yells Peter. "Mommy fik-its!" And I
hear his bare feet stamping out a tattoo of distress on the
floorboards.

"Coming!" I yell back almost cheerfully.

Easter baskets, woven of brightly colored construction
paper and stuffed with tangles of bilious-green tissue-paper

grass and with pastel eggs, hang from the corridor walls of the children's ward at Columbia Presbyterian Hospital. Some of the Scotch tape has curled away from the wall. The decorations flap in the breeze each time the automatic double doors swing open like fans, across a black rubber mat, activated by a footfall or the pressure of a stretcher from the operating room or a wheelchair from the patient's lounge.

"Where's Peter?" says Larry.

"Peter should be coming down from OR any minute now," says Dr. Tierney. "We had quite a time with your young fellow."

"What do you mean?" I ask, suddenly frightened.

"Oh, nothing serious. Last night one of the nurses found him standing in front of the elevator with his suitcase. He had managed to pack his bag and climb out of his crib. He's quite a little tiger. Luckily, she caught him, or he'd be wandering around 168th Street wearing nothing but a wrist tag and a diaper!"

"How did he react to the tests?" Larry asks, man to man.

"Well, we ran into some minor difficulties there, too. Peter had what we call a paradoxical reaction to phenobarbital. Instead of putting him to sleep, the phenobarb agitated him. Paradoxical reactions are really quite common. We've noted it on his chart. That way, if he ever needs some more tests, they'll know to use another sedative."

An Easter basket flutters on the wall.

"Ah! Here comes the little rebel now," says Dr. Tierney as the doors swing open. "Naturally, he's still a bit dopey."

I catch a glimpse of Peter being pushed out of the elevator and down the hall in a wheelchair. I am all ready to call out, Hi, old bean, old sock, old Fudgetickle Entworth LaRue, old Flutter Bottom Thumb Sucker the Third, but I can't speak. Peter sits slumped, pale, staring into space. I have seen those bewildered, ominous eyes before. They are eyes that have seen the worst, the eyes of the Holocaust children.

I do not dare to ask the questions that suddenly line up in my mind, clamoring, rowdy, shoving against one another to be heard. Are you saying that he felt the needles of the electromyogram penetrating deep into the muscle tissue of his arms and legs? And, do you mean—oh my God—do you mean that he may have felt the scalpel cutting through the muscles of his calf? And, does he hate me for letting this happen to him? And, what have I done? Why have I let these doctors take a two-inch slice from the muscle of my baby's leg just to satisfy themselves, with scientific exactitude, that he does, indeed, have the very dystrophy, Duchenne type, that they were confident he had all along?

My mind is on the rampage, stamping, kicking, screaming, roughing me up until I admit the truth. I didn't want to think about this. I don't want to be responsible for this. I don't want to take care of a dying child.

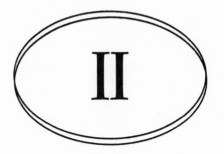

II

"What was it that I used to think about?" I say to Larry, who has just stopped reading next to me in bed where I am unraveling a piece of dental floss.

"I don't know," he answers, eyes staring, unfocused, at a place on the opposite wall.

"I don't mean that I think about it *all* the time, but I think about it so much that I can't imagine what thoughts this new thought has replaced."

"I know exactly what you mean," says Larry flatly, trancelike.

"It is as if, for the past two years, there is this new place in me, or at least a new feeling. Sometimes it feels like a fist clenched in my gut, and sometimes it feels like an ache, a hole punched out in the center of me, an absence in me. It is where I return to when the music stops. I mean, if the doorbell rings, I jump up to open the door and my mind is filled with thoughts coming alive, taking wing. Maybe it's the mailman with something too big to fit into the mailbox, maybe it's a present that's too early for somebody's birthday, and sometimes I imagine that it's Mr. Anthony from John Beresford Tipton calling to hand us a check for a million dollars, but whoever it turns out to be, as soon as I shut the door and the event is over, my thoughts flutter weakly and sink of their own weight down into that hole. It is home to me. It is where I wake up in the morning. Oh, Larry, do you think we will ever get used to this?"

"Maybe we should have another child." Larry reaches over to pat me on the stomach.

The skin on my belly spasms. "We don't even feel like fucking, so how are we going to make a baby, never mind a female baby?"

"It might help," says Larry, his face furrowing into an expression of contempt, "if you would stop flossing your teeth. It's not much of a turn-on."

"Waiting while you make neat piles of change on the bed-side table is hardly an aphrodisiac."

"Mary-Lou, the truth is that you haven't felt like making love since we learned about Peter."

"And the truth is that you are a selfish coward. You are delighted to be an overworked lawyer and a real pal to Adam so that you'll be too busy, or too tired, or too necessary to Adam's well-being, to be with me and Peter."

"For Chrissakes, I'm with you two whenever I have a free moment!"

"That's just the point. You make sure that you have damn few of them."

"What the hell do you want from me? I work my ass off all day, and when I finally get home I want to relax. And, as a matter of fact, I think Adam needs extra attention from his father." Larry says the last words, "extra attention from his father," in a tone of voice that suggests worse than rectitude.

"Perfect!" I mock. "Just perfect! Poor overworked Daddy comes home to find his older son craving the love and attention that he should be getting from his Mother, but, alas, she's *so* doting, *so* overinvolved with the younger child, simply because he's dying, that she doesn't have much time to spend with her first child." Now I am really screaming. Tears of fury and frustration trace down my enflamed cheeks. I feel ugly.

"Mary-Lou, I just can't talk to you when you're like this. I think you say things you don't mean. I really don't want to take this conversation any further."

"This isn't a conversation, you fucker, this is an argument. And I am saying exactly what I mean. What I mean is that I am furious with you. What I mean is that I feel all alone. What I mean is I feel gypped. What I mean is that I feel as if Adam is becoming your child, and that Peter is all mine— my problem, my sorrow, my fault!"

"Come on! What do you mean 'my problem, my sorrow, my fault'? What's the matter with you! What do you suppose I am thinking about all day? You don't suppose I think about much else, do you, you tragedy queen." Larry's voice rasps: " 'Your honor,' I sometimes want to say in open court, 'may it please the court, my son is dying!' " His voice breaks, and I see him cry for the second time, those blips and whimpers, the poignant incongruity of a little boy's runny nose on a grown man's upper lip.

"Hey, Larry," I say softly, dabbing at his tears with the edge of the sheet, "I'm sorry. I know you hurt as much as I do. I'm sorry. That was a lousy thing for me to say. It's just that you never seem sad. You always seem so energetic, so in control."

"I feel helpless, impotent. Ol' Daddy no can fik-its," says Larry, backing away from despair. "It's all an act. It may fool you, but it doesn't fool me."

"Please don't pretend to be okay, okay?" I stroke the fine black hairs that tangle across the back of his hand, as if to tame him. "Because I *do* get fooled. You fool me every time. I actually believe that you're fine, and then I feel all alone."

Larry laces his fingers through mine and lifts my hand to

his lips. "I'll try," he says, grazing my knuckles with soft, dry kisses. "I'll try to keep you better cumps."

"Thanks. Sometimes I feel so lonely." I tie the ends of the dental floss together and tug on them smartly to be sure. Then I slip my hands inside and separate them as far apart as they can be, the way I used to hold the yarn for Mother.

"Your mother lives ten minutes away in Fairfield; your father lives ten minutes away in Westport. You'd think . . . you'd think they'd try to help you in some—"

"Yes," I interrupt. "You would." I don't want to get started. I don't want to add fury to sorrow.

"At least you've got Glenny. What about Glenda the Good?"

"She's a good friend, and she's good company, too," I allow, "but you're the only person who can keep me company where I am."

"Where are you?"

"Up shit creek. You are Peter's only other parent." I scoop up the waxy string from my left palm with the middle finger of my right hand, and discover myself playing cat's cradle.

"Do you think you'd feel less lonely, less sad, if we had a baby?"

"I don't know. I think about it a lot, ever since we got the results of my biopsies from the geneticist." I examine the triangular wedges of string, taut between my hands. "Sometimes I think 'yes,' and sometimes 'no.' When it's 'yes,' I feel disloyal to Pete, somehow, as if we were already replacing him, phasing him out . . . and when I think 'no,' I betray my own instincts to thrive." With the middle finger of my left hand, I scoop up the string from my right palm. Two flexible X's, perfect for the picking, stretch between my palms. This is as far as I can go alone.

"You sure don't make life easy for yourself, do you?" Larry's voice sounds teasing, chiding, but I can tell he's pissed. "You've got things prearranged in your head so that no matter what you do, you're fucked. That's a kind of arrogance, you know."

"*What's* a kind of arrogance?"

"Being so sure that everything's going to turn out wrong. Your pessimism."

"You may be right," I mumble. I present him with the cat's cradle. "Go ahead; it's your turn."

"I've forgotten how to do it."

"You just pinch it here and here." I point with my chin. "Go ahead."

Larry's fingers descend, pinch, lift and fumble and the floss goes slack, like a broken web. "Abracadabra!" he cheers weakly.

"Maybe it would be a good idea."

"What?"

"To have a baby. I'd love to have a little girl. What a wonderful time in history it is to have a female child!"

"I'd love it too," says Larry.

"Well, if we're going to do it, we'd better do it soon, before Peter's care gets too preoccupying."

"Are you willing to take a chance? It's our baby, but it's your pregnancy, and if it's a boy, it'll be your abortion. I really think we've got to be very sure we know what we're doing."

"I really think it's a good idea. Actually, it's better than a good idea. It's a lifesaver of an idea. A baby would feel good. A baby would be more life, instead of less. Someone growing. Someone for Peter to be bigger than, and smarter than."

"Someone else for Adam to love, besides Pete," Larry adds.

"Someone for us all to love."

"Let's fuck!"

"Remember what Dr. Kittenplan said!"

"Did he say 'Let's fuck' too?"

"No, idiot. He said to 'think girl.' "

"Does it help to have your socks off or on?"

"Dr. Landrum B. Shettles—he's the guy who wrote a book about how you can choose the sex of your baby—recommends a vinegar douche, to make the vaginal environment less hospitable to male-making sperm." I pronounce each word with a hoity-toity flourish.

"An odd name."

"You think Landrum B. Shettles is an odd name, just wait till I tell you the name of the guy who performs the amniocentesis."

"I'm waiting."

"Dr. Cherry!"

"It'll be nice to know," says Larry wryly, "that each and every time we make love, Doctors Kittenplan, Shettles and Cherry will be in bed with us, cheering us on, giving me performance anxiety."

Do they "do it," I wonder. Do my parents "do it"?

Desperate, like some ratiocinative detective, I begin to search the house for clues of love. No smells of warm loaves cooling waft love from the kitchen. A once-gouged Jell-O aspic with little carrot scrapings magically suspended in it trembles on a refrigerator shelf. Chocolate pudding shrinks away from the sides of Pyrex custard cups, its leathery skin dense and shiny.

There must be some love around here somewhere. There has to be. Parents and children live here, after all. I go looking for evidence. Somebody must be giving some. Somebody must be getting some.

I look in the bathroom. I forage feverishly in the mirrored medicine cabinet, discarding cold cream, pancake make-up, aspirin, Chen Yu nail polish and cotton balls. At last I come upon a tiny, flat, round container of whitish cream. Stuck to the lid, a yellowed prescription label reads: "Herbert Louis Cohen. Apply nightly to affected area."

There it is. Evidence. They do "do it." Nightly. The man inserts his penis into the woman's vagina and fertilizes the egg. This happens when two people are married and very much in love. Nightly. According to prescription. Nightly the cream is applied by Herbert Louis Cohen to the affected area, and it is dark and Herbert Louis Cohen inserts his penis into the vagina of Gertrude Mary Cohen and fertilizes the egg that makes Mary-Lou Cohen and they are married and very much in love.

I try very hard to imagine this. It is impossible. It is more impossible even than imagining my science teacher, Mr. Pjura, "doing it" to my social studies teacher, Miss Falkowski. It is more impossible and not nearly as funny. I do not believe for a minute that my parents do this. My father reads the Times, *tees off at the country club, plays late Beethoven quartets, smokes Parliaments, wins cases, and says, "In the final analysis." He does not insert anything into anything.*

"First of all, let us review what we have learned from our genetic detective work," says Dr. Kittenplan eagerly, getting up from behind the desk, his nimble, wiry frame unfolding with the jerky levity of a marionette.

I can see that he loves his work.

Dr. Kittenplan slides a piece of chalk out from the ledge below his office blackboard, which is green. Rolling a stub of chalk between his palms, he continues, "We know from the maternal history that your sister's male child is unaffected, that your mother's brother and his son are also unaffected, and that your mother's younger sister has two adopted children. Correct?" He pauses, his right hand poised at the top of the blackboard, his head turned sharply over his left shoulder. He is making sure that he has our attention. I meet his gaze with unwavering fidelity. I am an eager learner. I can feel the answer fluttering against my ribs. I just know I am right. I am sure that I am all right.

"Furthermore," Dr. Kittenplan intones through the black wiry hairs in his nose, "we have the evidence that you, Mrs. Weisman, probably are not a carrier. We base this on the negative results on all three tests—the blood serum, the muscle biopsies and the electromyogram. Then, of course, there is the additional information that your older son, Adam, I believe his name is, is normal."

I can hardly keep from laughing out loud. I am not a carrier! I am not a carrier! I knew it! I just knew it! The unspoken words bounce for joy up and down in my brain.

"Unfortunately," Dr. Kittenplan croons on in his second-generation inflection, a blend of Bronx glottal and Talmudic singsong, "these tests cannot prove conclusively that you are *not* a carrier, although they can, in about seventy percent of those tested, prove that you are."

"I don't think I understand what you just said," I say, stunned.

"Let me put it another way." The doctor places his palms together and presses the sides of his index fingers against his pursed lips. "The tests failed to prove that you were a carrier, but the tests are only about seventy percent accurate."

"You mean," I recite back numbly, "I still might be a carrier."

"Exactly." Dr. Kittenplan is satisfied that I understand. "However," he adds, "the likelihood is that you are not. In fact," he pronounces, writing with a squeaky flourish on the blackboard, "I have calculated the odds. The statistical odds of a pregnancy of yours resulting in another male baby with Duchenne dystrophy are one in forty."

I stare at the chalk child on the blackboard.

"Peter." I hear my own voice speaking. "Peter."

"What?" says Dr. Kittenplan.

"Peter is the one. Peter is the one in forty." I struggle to explain what I have just understood myself. "Your statistic is Peter," I finally blurt out. "One in forty looks like good odds in chalk, but in real life it's much too much. One in one hundred is too much. Any possibility of any more is too much."

"Well, of course," says Dr. Kittenplan, tossing the chalk impatiently from hand to hand, "all I can do is work out the odds based on all the available information. Naturally, you must come to your own decision. I would not presume to advise you about that, except to say that were you to become pregnant with a female, the chances are also one in forty that she would be a carrier, although she would not have the disease."

"Then it's settled," I say. "If I'm pregnant with a male, I will get an abortion."

"Or," adds Dr. Kittenplan, "if it's a male, at least you

know what the odds are. When you're gambling, it's helpful to know what the odds are."

"I'm not going to gamble, Dr. Kittenplan."

"Well, of course, that's your decision," he says with professional rectitude.

"I'm not going to gamble because I can't afford to lose."

"Then I suggest you tell your husband to think girl." He smiles unprofessionally as he ushers me out of his office.

There is an insubstantial smudge of harvest moon still visible in the morning sky, like a daub of flour on a Wedgwood plate. Standing under the morning moon, waiting for Larry to back the car out of the garage, I look down at myself and wonder if it shows.

"Sixteen weeks," Dr. Kittenplan had said. "You have to wait sixteen weeks before it is safe to take enough amniotic fluid to sex the cells which have been sloughed off by the developing fetus."

"Oh God, please, God," I say out loud, under the sky, placing my hands, palms down, on either side of my belly, "make it a girl. I don't know why you should do anything for me, since I don't even believe in you, and I can't even honestly say I promise to believe in you if the baby is a girl. But if you really exist, this is the sort of thing you should be doing gratis. I mean, if you can be God for someone like me who doesn't even believe in you and probably isn't ever going to, no matter what, just think how genuinely godly an act that would be. It's really a perfect, godly sort of thing to recognize me, even if I don't recognize you, to love me, even when I don't love you. I mean, at least I'm honest. At least give me credit for not being a hypocrite. Amen."

We ride toward New York City in absolute silence. There is nothing to say that will not open abruptly upon a defeat too painful to invite prematurely, or a victory too wonderful to be trifled with in anticipation. Terror and hope close together like a vise in my chest. Time is standing still.

* * *

Except for a Sabrett hot-dog cart and a bag lady mumbling into a litter can, nobody seems to be in our part of Central Park this brisk and azure September morning.

"Would you like a hot dog?" says Larry.

"It's not even eleven o'clock," I answer.

"I didn't ask you for a time check, I asked if you want a hot dog."

"No thank you. I do not care for a hot dog at this particular moment."

"Try to relax. You're awfully nervous," says Larry. "It's like waiting for the jury to come in."

"It's worse. At least with a jury, how well you do has something to do with the outcome. We have no control. We are, as they say, at the mercy of the fates. How long have we been waiting here, anyway?"

"Almost two hours."

"Jeezus."

Two interns rush by, their tangled stethoscopes stuffed, with what I am sure is studied carelessness, into the starched pockets of their white lab jackets.

"Those are just the kind of men my mother wanted me to marry."

"You mean doctors?"

"I mean Jewish doctors."

"How can you tell they're Jewish?"

"I read their names on the tags they were wearing."

"For Chrissakes, Mary-Lou, you're incredible. They went by so quickly. Why did you bother to read their names?"

"The same reason a chicken crosses the road, silly. To see if they're Jewish. Want to know what else I know?"

"What else?"

"I know how big their cocks are."

"Really?" Larry yelps. "Jeezus! I don't believe it. Okay, go ahead, tell me. How big *are* their cocks?"

"Well," I drawl, warming to the task, "the one nearest to Fifth Avenue, H. Silverman, M.D., has a big one."

"How can you tell?"

"Well, first I check out their hands. If their hands are particularly big, and their fingers particularly thick, the chances are eight out of ten that they will have big cocks. Then I confirm my diagnosis by checking out the size of the bulge in their pants, or, in the more challenging instance of boxer shorts, the faint outline of the glans visible either on the left or the right inseam. H. Silverman, for instance, wears boxer shorts."

"Jeezus!"

"On the other hand, M. Goldberg, M.D., has a small one and wears Jockey shorts. Actually, I think H. Silverman would be more comfortable if he wore Jockey shorts like M. Goldberg."

"Maybe you should tell him."

"Mebbe I will if he walks by again."

"Oh, M'Lou, M'Lou," Larry chides, taking my hands and pressing them tightly between his, "I love you. You're nuts, but I love you."

"I love you too," I say. "What time is it?"

"A couple of minutes later than it was the last time you asked."

"How time flies when you're having fun. Someday I hope we're going to laugh about this. Kee-rist, I sound like a soap opera. What the hell, this *is* like a soap opera. I mean, really, how much soapier can you get? There I am, flat on my back, belly up, while Dr. you-should-pardon-the-expression Cherry, needle in hand, says, 'Don't worry. I haven't missed yet.'—And the mad dash from Ninety-second and Park over to Kittenplan's lab with a test tube full of amniotic fluid in your vest pocket. Remember all the temperature-taking with the Ovatherm and the vinegar douches?" I elbow his ribs, nudging him away from sobriety. "And the time you said, 'Would Madame like the house dressing this evening?' Actually, it's too silly to be a soap opera. It's a soap opera starring the Marx Brothers." My voice sounds wild and giddy, even to me. "What time is it, Larry?" I ask, unable to endure myself in silence either.

"A little after eleven."

"Larry?" I pause to make sure that I have snagged him on my conversational hook.

"Yes?"

"I have a deep-down feeling that it's going to be a girl. It's our turn to get lucky. I know it. Don't you think so?"

"I know I love you," Larry murmurs, tilting his face near mine, nibbling at my lips.

"I love you too," I say between little kisses.

Out of the corner of my eye I see Dr. Kittenplan waving to us as prearranged from across Fifth Avenue. He looks like a tailor masquerading as a doctor. His slightly concave chest suggests piecework performed in a bent-over position.

It is impossible to tell from the look on his face whether he has good news or bad. We follow him down the hospital corridors, turning right or left each time we come face to face with a wall. I look for clues in the creases where his starched white jacket strains across his shoulder blades. I try to read messages in the room numbers as we pass, to draw meaning from the glimpse of a nurse filing her nails in the linen room.

I wager that the elevator will come before I can count to ten. That Dr. Kittenplan will step into the elevator before Larry. That the elevator won't stop on any other floor but ours.

"If I can hold my breath until the eighth floor. If Larry gets out of the elevator before Dr. Kittenplan. If I don't step on a crack and break my mother's back. If his office door is open. If the number has more than two digits. If there is any love or mercy in this world for us, please let it be a girl." I finally allow the words to form and come together in my brain as Dr. Kittenplan ushers us into his office.

"I'm sorry I kept you waiting so long," he says. "We wanted to check and double-check the results. We sexed several different cells, and they all have male sex chromosomes. I'm sorry. You may look for yourself," he says, smiling and inclining his head, bowing at the waist a bit, gesturing toward his microscope with an open, almost flourishing palm, inviting me to inspect it for myself, just to make sure there has been no funny business. It is as if he were a magician and I a representative from the audience. He has selected me to go up onstage with him and bear witness to his amazing feat. I have been chosen to inspect close up, as close as I care to get, as close as I dare to get, to look inside the hat, to pick it up, turn it over, even to tap it with his magic stick, the one that just a moment ago had all the different-colored, knotted-together silk handkerchiefs stuffed all the way into it.

I step up and dutifully, dumbly, lower my face toward the microscope. Tears form, distorting my vision and threatening to overwhelm and splash into the eyepiece.

"Do you see the nucleus of the cell, Mary-Lou? It should appear red and granular. Have you located it?" I hear Dr. Kittenplan's words through the aching, echoing sorrow that is tolling inside my head.

"Yes," I answer, seeing something transparent and oval, like a tear.

"If the cell were from a female fetus, you would see a darker, denser, triangular shape called a Barr body against the wall of the nucleus," Dr. Kittenplan says over my shoulder, adding, "Perhaps you'd like to take a look too, Larry."

I do not want to give up my place. I do not want to lift my face up from the microscope. If only time would stand still. If only I could be enchanted in this spot, hidden and protected in this moment between sentencing and execution.

I feel the weight of Larry's arm across my shoulders and the scrape of his tweed sleeve against my cheek. He does not pause to take a look for himself. Instead, he leads me away from the microscope, past Dr. Kittenplan, out of his office, down the elevator, through the hospital corridors, and back into the park.

"We've been giving a lot of thought to adopting a baby, Mom."

Sitting with Mother at the kitchen table, I roll the salt shaker back and forth between my palms and stare down at the holes on top.

Tick. Tick. Tick. The tiny metallic tick, tick, tick of Mother's knitting needles as they touch and slide, touch and slide, is her only response.

"An infant. An infant so that we can be reasonably sure that it hasn't been mistreated in a foster home or something."

Only the ticking of her needles and the satiny whoosh of her breathing.

"And of course we'd work through a reputable agency, a Jewish one. Like the Louise Wise or whatever," I keep talking.

Tick. Tick. Tick. More. She wants more. Tell her more.

"I don't think I could stand another abortion. When the doctor injected the saline solution into my womb, I felt life. I felt the baby die. It was awful!"

Tick. Tick. Tick. I don't dare to look up from the salt and into her face, and find no comfort there.

"I don't know exactly why it is, but I'm afraid to adopt. I don't want someone else's children. I want *our* children. I sound like a terrible snob, I know. I *am* a snob. I don't know if I could love an adopted child as much as my own. I'm ashamed of feeling that way. I don't want to feel that way. But I do." I roll the glass shaker back and forth, feeling the bevels press into my palms. "I wish I could overcome that. Just when I'm on the verge of deciding 'yes,' I lose heart. And yet I want a baby so much!" I set the shaker down on the table and look up. "What do you think, Mom?"

"Well, dear . . ." Mother's fingers stop their frantic conjuring. She crosses her needles, midair, in the rest position. "It's true, when you adopt, you never know what you're going to get. You can't trust any agency to check the backgrounds thoroughly enough. Do you remember the Brody child? She was the prettiest infant I had ever seen." Mother smiles at the thought of the Brody baby. "Not a mark on her. She must have been a Caesarean.

"In any case, she turned out to be damaged goods. Subnormal. Imagine how those parents felt!" Mother gives a yank on the yarn and the whole ball of wool flies out of her handbag and rolls across the kitchen floor. "Get that for me, will you, dear?"

"I suppose you're right, Mother." I get up as instructed and retrieve the ball. "You never do know what you're going to get." It doesn't seem to matter to me in the slightest, except, perhaps as irony, that Larry and I—a one-in-a-hundred red-headed Caucasian *magna cum laude* and a tall, dark, handsome doctor of jurisprudence—that these two healthy specimens pooled their genes, mingled their marvelous backgrounds (especially hers) and created a child who was "damaged goods." I hand her the yarn.

"Thank you, dear." The needles begin to move again. I watch her index finger dive and stab at the air and come up garroted by a loop of yarn which it then feeds to the waiting needle. "By the way, dear, are you absolutely sure that Peter has multiple sclerosis?"

"Why do you ask?" I respond cautiously.

"Because I was at a cocktail party last night at the Simonses, you know, the Lester Simonses of New Rochelle? Well," she rushes on without waiting for any sign of recognition from me, "I met a very interesting young doctor there. Actually, he's an optometrist, but he's Jewish," she adds, as if being Jewish almost makes up for not being a real M.D. "Well," she says, "one thing led to another, and we somehow got to talking about terminally ill children. Of course, I told him about Peter's multiple sclerosis, and he said that while it wasn't exactly his field, he had never before heard of a child five years old having multiple sclerosis."

"That's because Peter has muscular dystrophy," I answer flatly, impassively.

"Oh, dear," Mother says, "I must have gotten the disease wrong."

"Five sinks. *Five* fucking sinks. Who would ever have thought that someday I'd own *five sinks*? Jeezus! I never even wanted one!" Larry rips the check out of the checkbook and slips it in the envelope. "To Tom Duffy, plumber, sixty-three dollars."

I can tell by the tone of his voice that he's whipping himself up into one of those I-work-my-fingers-to-the-bone fits. "Sixty-three's not so bad." I talk over the sound of running water.

"Mr. Weis-man, oh Mr. Weis-man," hollers the voice of a small child from the yard. "Mr. Wei-yi-yize-man," it concludes with a mournful yodel.

"For Chrissakes, who's calling me?" snarls Larry, getting up from the kitchen table, where he is paying bills. "Do you want to renew our subscription to *The New Yorker*?"

"It sounds like Freddie," I say, ripping off my aqua Playtex Living Gloves with surgical panache. I hang them over the faucet. Even though I wear rubber gloves to do the dishes, I still have eczema on my fingers. "Actually, I'm too busy to read it. I just look at the cartoons. Let's get it again."

"Why?"

"First of all, because I like the cartoons, and second of all, because I wish I had time to read it."

"I love the way your mind works." Larry opens the window. "What's the matter, Freddie?" he calls.

"Mr. Weis-man," he whines, "Adam said the f-word."

"Oh, fuck off, Freddie," Larry says out the window. "Christ, that kid gives me a swift pain in the ass."

"I hope he didn't hear you."

"Why? Are you afraid he's going to go home and tell his mommy on me?"

"*You* fuck off, Larry. You know, you're so goddamn hostile and uptight these days, you're impossible to live with."

"Nice, very nice. Most understanding. I really appreciate that from you." His voice is full of sarcasm, his face dark and furrowed with anger. "I exhaust myself all week in court and then I get to spend the whole weekend paying bills and watching Pete fall to his knees and bang the back of his head on the floor. And when I turn for a little comfort to my wife, she's 'too tired,' but that's not really much of a problem anymore since I can't come, anyway."

Suddenly the air is vacuous, sucked of voice and breath. The room is a coffin. I can feel words—some words, any words—urgently pounding at the back of my throat to be said, to fill the stifling void, but I do not know what they would say. We stand accused, accusing. We turn toward, and on, each other. We are each other's alibi.

I cast my eyes downward, looking for something to see besides the pain and fury in my husband's eyes. A letter, crisp and white, the business size, lies open on its back on the kitchen table, among the bills.

Dear Mr. Weisman:

Thank you for your letter of inquiry. Unfortunately, at present, neither the Yale Law School nor the Yale School of Medicine offers scholarships to lawyers who wish to matriculate into medical school. However, we wish you every success with what appears to be an exciting and ambitious pursuit.

"Larry?"

"What."

"What's this letter from Yale about?"

"Oh, *that.*" Larry offhandedly flicks the backs of his fingers at the letter's edge, sending it spinning. "That was just a crazy idea I had a while ago."

"Maybe it was a good crazy idea. Maybe it would help." I evoke the euphemistic "help" that we seem to have agreed upon in some solemn, silent pact is to stand for the unspeakable and constant low-grade pain each of us feels.

"It's a moot point, anyway." Larry reaches for the checkbook. "With this new house, I can't afford to do anything but what I've been doing for the past seven years." He opens the black vinyl-covered book and flips through the torn, serrated pages, jagged as shark's teeth. Oh shit. He is going to do a reading.

"How much do I owe them?" he begins. "Let me count the ways. To builder Tom Shaw, for renovations to ranch house, thirty-five thou, and that's not counting the base purchase price of thirty-eight thou."

He flips more and more pages brusquely, hitting his stride. "Hardly any deposits. Just withdrawals, withdrawals, withdrawals. I'm surprised the ink isn't running red. I'm hemorrhaging! Cash flow, my ass! To Scott Pools—wait a second . . . hold it . . . forgive me—to Scott *Aquascapes,* for swimming pool, sixteen thou. And that's just the aqua part. We haven't gotten to the scapes yet. The landscaping, including the hexagonal redwood deck, the flagstone ramp, naturalistic granite outcroppings and perpetually blooming plants, amounts to another four thou." He scowls up from his reading like a lawyer—rectitude triumphant.

"You were the one who said, 'If we're going to do it, let's do it right,'" I say. "You were the one who didn't want the pool to look like a HoJo motor lodge, surrounded by concrete and a chain-link fence, for Chrissakes."

"I never said it had to be so goddamn naturalistic that the fucking ducks use it for a toilet on their way south!"

"Don't be a schmuck, Larry. The pool was a great idea and you know it. Pete loves the pool. He feels so buoyant in the water. He can do things in the water that he can't do on land anymore. Can you imagine what a treat so little gravity must be for him! Whatever the price, it's worth it. And I'm glad it's beautiful. I've got a feeling we're going to be putting in a lot of time around here. Maybe the best years of our lives, whenever they're supposed to start . . ."

"I think they're the ones that just ended," Larry interjects. "You know it's not the money. I don't really mind the money. I want Peter to have everything we can possibly afford. I'd steal for him gladly."

"You'd die for him."

"Yes."

"The problem is that there's nothing that you can do, darling, and you're a do-er."

"A no-can-do-er."

"Think of it this way: you proved that money can buy happiness. You should have seen him this aft, Larry." I hear my voice. It swells with motherly brag. "I put one of the wrought-iron porch chairs into the shallow end of the pool, and Pete had the best time just getting in and out of it! He's got a game going. He assumes a seated position in the water and just allows himself to float gently down into the chair. Then, when he's ready to come back up for a breath, he just presses down lightly on the arm rests with his fingers, and up he bounces. You wouldn't believe the way he was grinning when his face broke the surface of the water. And then he yelled, 'Ta-daa! Ladies and gentlemen, ta-daa!'" We both laugh out loud like two proud parents.

For a silent moment we stand at the window, leaning against each other, watching Peter, Adam and Freddie play. The backyard is cluttered with toppled tricycles and croquet mallets, the evidence of short attention spans. An early autumnal wind blows, pocking the surface of the pool with shivers. Overhead, two mallards flying by shift their wings into reverse and beat them frantically while they descend toward the water in a downward skid, their webbed feet angled for landing.

We hear Peter's squeaky voice trilling across the yard and through the open window. "Look-it how fast I can run! Look-it, Freddie. Look-it, Adam. Look-it!"

I feel a familiar stab in my gut, like falling in a dream.

"Betcha I can beatcha, betcha," Freddie challenges.

"Look-it," pipes Peter, and I can see without looking that his fists are clenched as tightly as he can clench them, that he is thrusting his little shoulders forward, urging his legs to follow their example, and I know that his movement is so arduous, so slow, that even his fine, silken hair is unruffled.

"See?" Peter says proudly. "See how fast?"

"That's not fast," says Freddie. "That's slow."

"It's pretty fast," we hear Adam say.

"Please take a seat, Mrs. Weisman. Doctor will be with you shortly." The nurse pronounces "Doctor" the way a nun says "Father," in the worshipful familiar.

I take a seat in Dr. Tierney's empty office. "Doctor will be with you shortly my ass," mumbles the dybbuk warming up inside my brain. I can see Dr. Tierney darting in and out of the corridor doorways, visiting patients, like a hotly pursued lover in a bedroom farce.

Seated in the soft leather chair facing his desk, I feel chilly, impatient, tender, as if I were perched on a hard enamel stool wrapped in a stiff white paper angel gown, bound at the waist by a string of white plastic rickrack, offering up my warm urine in a cold steel bowl.

I get up and begin to roam his tiny office, inspecting the seams of the wallpaper and staring at the white-and-brown marbelized vinyl floor until I remember that what it reminds me of is halvah. I pause at his scale long enough to weigh my shoes. Still no doctor.

I lift the glass lid off the cotton-ball container, grab some and stuff them deep into my coat pocket. I swipe a tongue depressor—for Peter, I tell myself—and stuff it in, too.

Emboldened, my larcenous fingers creep toward the file marked "Peter Weisman," which lies closed on Tierney's desk, and snatch it, searching for secrets.

My eyes rummage feverishly through the pages, translating intriguing clusters of numbers into November 2, 1964— Peter's birthday, for Chrissakes.

What is this word here, scrawled in the mysterious hieroglyphs of medicine, full of consonants from the Greek? It's "dystrophic." Of course. Still, I examine it closely as if it were a code and I, by sorting out the letters, might break it and find the cure.

In fact, I learn what I already know. Every six months,

when we take Peter to see Tierney, we learn what we already know. Dr. Tierney is in charge of watching Peter die. These are his notes—a nihilist's journal.

I close the file and get out from behind the desk. Just in time.

"Good morning, Mary-Lou. I hope I haven't kept you waiting too long," says Dr. Tierney, smiling and extending his hand. "I did my very best to fit you in."

"No, not long, not long at all," I murmur, aware that the proximity of a doctor, like falling in love, makes me feel shy and virginal. Something tentative inside me dilates, expectant, hopeful.

He looks at me with his certain blue eyes and tells me that he has discovered the cure for muscular dystrophy in time to save Peter while he is still just barely walking.

I take a small, hesitant step or two toward him. I plan merely to express my gratitude. He must never know how much I love him.

Suddenly I am in his arms. He tilts my face upward and studies me with the look of love. He presses his lips against mine, sending a galvanic shiver of sweetness through my loins. "Dr. Tierney!" I cry, clinging to him, trembling, "Dr. Tierney! Ah! Dr. Tierney!"

And afterward he says, "Mary-Lou, my dearest, you must call me Doctor. I have always loved you from that first moment I saw you. Since then, I have worked night and day to save your child, hardly daring to hope that I might also win your love."

"Doctor!" I cry with perfect happiness. "Ah! Doctor!"

"So what can I do for you today, Mary-Lou?" Dr. Tierney lowers his large frame into his reclining leather desk chair.

Cure Peter. That's what you can do, squawks the dybbuk. "I just want to let you know," I say, "that Larry and I have made up our minds about the heel-cord operation. We don't want Peter to have it." I look intently into Tierney's eyes, searching for a flinch of disapproval, a gleam of agreement. His eyes tell me nothing. They are wide open and mute as a Greek statue's.

"You're sure?" he asks, giving nothing away.

"It's not the kind of decision we could ever be sure of. It's not the kind of decision people ought to have to make. 'Render therefore unto Caesar the things which are Caesar's . . .' This one is clearly in God's department."

"So did you ask Him?" Dr. Tierney pauses for a moment before pronouncing the word "him," as if uncertain about whether or not it should be capitalized.

"He didn't answer," I say, and then, as casually as I can, I try to slip past his professional defenses. "What would you do if you were in our place?"

"Contrary to popular opinion," says Dr. Tierney, smiling at his Michelangelo hands, which rest, huge and patient, on top of Peter's file, "I'm not eager to play God myself." He looks up at me. "But if you think it might help you, I'll play the devil's advocate."

"Okay. I'd appreciate that." I sit up straight in my chair.

Dr. Tierney leans back, relaxed. The chair screams. "I wonder if you realize that by your decision, people will accuse you of hastening the time when Peter will be in a wheelchair, perhaps by as much as two years? That's two years when he might have been able to play more normally with his friends, two more years of relative independence."

I am ready with a response. Larry and I have played this game before. "But in order to gain those two years of walking, he has to endure an operation under total anesthesia in which his Achilles tendons are cut so that his heels can reach to the floor, then six weeks in plaster casts, and then, even then, he will only be able to walk, if 'walk' you can call it, stiff-legged in metal braces that reach to the tops of his thighs. And he might not get as much as a two-year reprieve. You said so yourself. It might be one year, or even less. It doesn't sound like a good deal to me. It sounds more like a Faustian bargain. Besides, I'm not sure that normalcy and independence are appropriate goals for Peter. No matter what we decide, Peter will be abnormal and dependent sooner or later."

"Sooner or later," Tierney repeats, lounging in his chair. "You are choosing to make it sooner. You are not even putting up a fight."

"It's the wrong fight." I rest my arms on his desk and lean forward. "Peter is so obsessed with his weakening muscles that he does nothing all day but challenge other kids to races that he keeps losing. He's five years old, and he shows no interest in reading. He won't even play. All he wants to do is keep moving. He's got all his energies, all his hopes, his whole sense of himself tied up in that. I don't feel right conspiring with him when I know better, when I know what's coming. All you're doing is fending off the inevitable and making it even harder to accept when it comes."

Tierney shifts his huge frame into a more upright position and picks up a pencil from his desk. First he presses the point into the blotter, anchoring it. Then, starting at the eraser end, he slides his thumb and forefinger slowly down the pencil's beveled sides. When his fingers reach the bottom, he turns the pencil over like an hourglass and repeats the procedure, this time from point to eraser. " 'Fending off the inevitable,' you say. Isn't that really all we are doing? Isn't time all any one of us has?"

"It's a part of what we've all got more or less of, but it's not all we've got. What we've decided is that Peter's life can't be about anything that happens over time. It can't be about when he can ride a two-wheeler, or a ten-speed; or about when he gets his driver's license, or into Harvard, or married, or successful. His life has to be about quality— about how well, how deep, how rich—not about how fast, how many, how soon, how long."

Dr. Tierney lounges back again and confides to the ceiling, "That sounds like a very high-minded philosophy. I wonder if it means anything? I wonder if she knows what she's talking about?"

"I wonder if it means anything too. I also wonder if she knows what she's talking about." I smile as the acid spill of irony curdles my evangelical soul. "You're right. I don't know what I'm talking about. I haven't the vaguest idea of how to love a child unconditionally, of how to bring up a child without expectations. I don't know how to live without expectations myself. Right now I can't even tell you what that life might be like. I can't even imagine it. But nevertheless, that's what we're committed to finding out. You're right. In the deepest sense of the words, I don't know what I'm talking about.

"All we know is that we are determined to find or make meaning in Peter's life, and that means that we must make some kind of peace, a peace I cannot now imagine, with the enemy, with the fact that an ever increasing part of Peter's life is his disease."

I grab the edge of Dr. Tierney's desk and lean forward. "Cure him! Cure him if you can! Go ahead! For God's sake, please." I withdraw my hands and settle back in my chair when I hear that I am almost screaming. "But you can't. I understand. Please keep on trying. But meanwhile, we've got to figure out how to live with the Peter who is, and we're just beginning to understand what that means. Horrible as it is, this is Peter's disease. It inhabits his cells. It flows in his blood. It is as much a part of his life as it will be his death. It must be respected. The disease has its integrity."

Dr. Tierney snaps upright in his chair. "Do you understand that your decision will have a direct bearing on the length of his life? The sooner he is in a wheelchair, the sooner his bones become brittle with disuse, and his respiration weak and shallow."

"I do."

"And you understand that you cannot change your mind in a couple of months? That this decision is irrevocable?"

"Yes."

"And you won't regret it when Peter's feet are so deformed that they won't fit into shoes?"

"Yes."

"Then," Dr. Tierney stands up behind his desk, extends his hand, and surrounds mine in a firm shake, "congratulations."

I scan his eyes once more, seeking the beam of agreement. I can't find it. "For what?"

"For holding your own against the devil's advocate."

"This can't be what I really want, can it?" says Larry to the tops of his wing-tip shoes as we walk through Greenwich Village in a fine, vaporous September rain. "We're on our way to having everything we ever thought we wanted out of life—"

"—and *then* some," I throw in for good measure. Lifestyle summations depress me.

"I'm talking about the factors we *can* control. A nice home, good friends, a terrific job, wonderful children, each other." He puts his arm around me and gives me a squeeze. "So why do I feel so lousy?"

"It's like Daddy's golf joke; you know, the one about the guy who's been an avid golfer all his life, the kind who neglects his wife and kids to play golf? Well, this son of a bitch dies and finds himself conversing with the Devil. The guy looks around and sees that he is standing on the first tee of what looks like the most challenging and well-kept golf course he has ever seen, and he is holding the nicest set of golf clubs he can imagine.

" 'Welcome to hell,' says the Devil warmly.

" 'This is hell?' says the golfer. 'This terrific golf course! These sensational clubs! If this is hell, I'm in heaven. C'mon,' he says to the Devil, 'let's tee off! What are we waiting for? Give me a ball and let's get going!'

" 'There are no balls,' says the Devil"—and here I pause a bit— " 'that's the hell of it.' "

"That's supposed to be funny?" Larry asks after a punishing silence.

"Not funny. Just pertinent," I explain. "This awful event has happened to us, this proverbial bolt from the blue, and nothing about our lives reflects the terrible change. We've gone on as if nothing has happened. There's something wrong with that. If we're going to have to endure the worst that life can deal us, why shouldn't we try to find the best life has to offer? Why batten down the hatches and sail out the storm? Why play it safe? Why not full speed ahead?" I bloat with hope. Oh Christ! I sound like Jane Froman playing Jane Froman.

"Maybe some kind of change would help," says Larry.

"Like what?"

"Like shipping out as stevedores, or maybe buying a farm."

"Adam gets seasick and I have hay fever."

"That reminds me," says Larry. "Keith Gilchrist called me at the office today. He wanted to know if we'd decided about going to the group in Bucks County with them."

"When is it? I forget."

"The weekend after next. We have to send in the registration fee right away if we want to go. Pennsylvania is beautiful in the fall."

"Do we want to go?"

"What are we doing, sharing a brain? What about *you*? Do you want to go?"

"I'm not sure. This encounter-group stuff sounds weird. The leader is somebody from Esalen. Nancy says they take their clothes off and yell at each other."

"That's not so weird. That's what we do every weekend too. We'll feel right at home."

I stop dead in my tracks and stare at my shoes. "Your jokes aren't so funny either."

"Why don't we just go!" Larry proposes, taking my hands. "We always have a good time with the Gilchrists. You'll love the Pennsylvania Dutch country. And besides, we're bummed out. We could both use a break. I'll call my mom, and if she and Eddie can come up and stay with the kids, we'll do it. Well"—he gives my fingers a little squeeze— "what do you say?"

I hesitate. Already my spirit feels the weight of the victim's inertia which grows like a hump on the back.

"C'mon!" Larry tugs at my hands playfully, but there is desperation in his eyes. "C'mon," he urges. "It might help."

"Sure. What the hell. Why not."

"Hey," Larry says suddenly, "look at the guy across the street!" He points to a black man walking swiftly alongside a couple.

"What's he doing?" I ask.

"He's panhandling. Watch his act, it's incredible. He's a real pro. Will you look at that! Watch him now. Watch what he does when he gets to the corner. See him? If he hasn't scored, he just pivots on one foot and picks up another victim on the backswing. Let's go over and talk to him."

"No, Larry. It's embarrassing!"

"Don't be such a coward. Let's just walk by and see what happens."

"I approaches you from the left," the panhandler says to Larry, slowing down to match our pace, "so as not to disturb the lovely young lady on your right. Would you be good enough, sir, to lend me thirty-seven cents?"

"Why thirty-seven cents?" asks Larry, more intrigued than ever.

"Because I already has the sixty-three cents, and a bottle of wine costiz a dollar."

"And if I give you the thirty-seven cents," says Larry in the sonorous, moralistic tones of white man's burden, "will you promise to stop panhandling on the street?"

"Hey, man," says the panhandler with the name "Gene" scripted on the top of his jacket pocket, "I ain't no panhandler. I just wants a loan."

"Aw, come on, Gene, you can't fool me. I've been watching your act from across the street. I bet you've already got enough change for ten bottles of wine."

"I already gots enough for twenty bottles," Gene replies smugly.

"Twenty bucks in small change!" Larry whispers, impressed. "How much do you make in a week?" He has suddenly dropped the burdensome tone.

"Well," says Gene, "I only works a two-day week, and even then I only works the night shiff. I makes about one hundred and fifty bucks on a good weekend."

"And what do you do the rest of the time?" Larry asks, delighted.

"Oh"—Gene shrugs toward the chain-linked cement playground across the street—"I plays checkers and I shoots baskets."

"Christ, man," exclaims Larry, getting downright comradely and colloquial, "you've got it made! You work two nights a week and make one hundred and fifty dollars, and the rest of the time you play checkers and shoot baskets? Shit, man, have you got it made!"

"I know I's got a good life," Gene answers thoughtfully. "But sometimes, specially around this time of year, I finds myself wondering, 'Is this what I really wants?' "

"No!" Betty Fuller shouts from a kneeling position as her fists hit the oversized pillow with a loud smack. Dust flies out from its paisley pores into the stale, smoky autumn air where it hangs like geometry in a shaft of sunlight. "No!" She is demonstrating how to get angry.

There are twelve other people in the Bucks County Seminar weekend workshop besides the Gilchrists and us, and not counting the leader, Betty, who is on loan from the Esalen Institute in Big Sur. Sixteen pairs of shoes stand in the corner—toes in, heels out—like little dunces sent there to atone. Like ballerinas at the barre, we've done all kinds of warm-ups, including a partners game called "Who are you?"

"Who are you?" the partner who is A asks the partner who is B. I am A. B smiles with shy anticipation and shakes the short brown curls, soft and glossy, that cover her head like a child's. Even though she is about my age, her pretty face glows with sheen and color, as if she'd just been towel-dried by an adoring mother.

We face each other, cross-legged, asking patiently over and over again like Indians, until we get the truth.

"Who are you?" I ask.

"Joyce."

"Thank you," I acknowledge, as I am supposed to. "Who are you?"

"Joyce Goodrich."

"Thank you. Who are you?"

"A psychologist." She cocks her head like a quick little bird listening for the worm.

"Thank you. Who are you?"

"A Ph.D." She smiles and then shrugs, as if she's discovered—just that second—that a Ph.D. is not what she'd meant to be, after all.

"Thank you. Who are you?"

"A seeker."

"Thank you. Who are you?"

"A meditator."

"Thank you. Who are you?"

"A wise, old woman."

"Thank you. Who are you?"

"A child."

"Thank you. Who are you?"

"A blind seeker."

"Okay, everybody," Betty yells. "Switch! A's become B's. B's become A's."

"Who are you?" Joyce asks.

"Mary-Lou."

"Thank you. Who are you?"

"Mary-Lou."

"Thank you. Who are you?"

"A wife."

"Thank you. Who are you?"

"A mother."

"Thank you. Who are you?"

"Mary-Lou."

Walter is a piece of brown rice. Susan is a crystal chandelier. Sally is a virus.

I am a holdout. If I could begin to tell the truth in this barn, resonant with time, its weathered walls dry and polished as bones picked bare by the truth, I would say that I am scared. Scared that all this nonsense might make sense. Scared that they, that I, might find me out for who I am.

"No!" Betty Fuller shouts once more, whipping her arched back forward as she struggles, over and over again, her long straight hair slapping, her face glistening like some great gray fish on a hook. "No! No! No!" she finishes.

Betty folds her voluptuously fat body back into the lotus position, touches her thumbs and middle fingers together and rests them daintily on her knees. Her underlying bony structure must be presumed; molten flesh pours over her like a drip castle.

Some terrific advertisement for mental health, I think to myself. No husband. No children. She must be at least forty. She must weigh at least two hundred and eighty. I imagine her eating Oreos in secret, raking away at the cream filling with her lower incisors. I imagine her trying to shave under her arms. I imagine her trying to "do it." I am sure she wishes she were married. I am sure she would settle for getting laid, this virgin Venus of Willendorf. I bring to bear all the prejudice and contempt an unhappy skeptic can muster against her considerable charisma.

"All right now, group, let's get to work," says Betty. "Everyone grab a pillow and pick a spot. Make sure there's plenty of room between you and the next guy."

Dutifully but reluctantly, I get up from the floor. I take one of the giant pillows and drag it by its ear toward a corner.

"Now, remember," Betty continues as sixteen people mill about, describing little circles and abandoning others in mid-curlicue, like dogs, each sensing, testing, seeking his perfect place in the room, "remember to keep breathing. You know, most people either breathe or do something. Rarely do you find someone who can breathe *and* do something at the same time. That's how we lock in our energy and drive ourselves crazy." She kneels in the center of the room in front of her demonstration pillow. "You can yell anything you want. I recommend that you start out by yelling 'No!' I find it works nicely as a general, all-purpose tantrum provoker. Maybe the 'No' will change into a 'Fuck you, Mom' or a 'Drop dead, Dad'—whatever. The important thing is to let the anger out. It will find its own focus and its own vocabulary.

"Okay, now. Everybody on all fours in front of a pillow. Put out the cigarette please, Joyce. Don't piss your anger away in smoke." Betty waits while Joyce puts out her cigarette and goes back to her pillow. "Okay?" She surveys the room from her knees, hands on her hips, a huge mother hen counting her chicks. "Everybody ready? Now let's get rid of some of that anger. Come on, ladies and gentlemen, get ready to give up a little of your beloved shit. Let's see you tight-asses let loose," she whoops like a general leading a charge. "Go sane!"

Not wanting to call attention to myself, my only alternative is to do it. Arms up, breathe in; arms down, breathe out, I say to myself as I arch my back and raise my clenched fists over my head and propel them downward into the pillow with a smooth, spinal whiplash.

"No!" I begin my obligatory tantrum. My "no" is an instant embarrassment, a powder puff tossed into a battlefield explosive with cannon-ball-sized noes. I yell louder, but my no-no-noes are swallowed up by the "shits" and "fucks" and "fuck yous" that now hurl through the air, spitting and sizzling like furious flares. The emotional ante is being upped. Can they really get so angry so fast? I hope they're full of shit, but I can't be absolutely sure.

"Fuck you!" I try out tentatively. Is "fuck you" the key to my private, primal animal kingdom? I decide to stick with "no."

"No!" I yell as my fists come down on the pillow. "No-o-o!" I bay like a hound.

"Mary-Lou." Betty is waddling over to me on her knees in a rocking side-to-side manner that causes her flowered mumu to stretch down taut over her abdomen. "You are holding back." Mother would disapprove of her outfit. Fat people should not wear large prints or horizontal stripes.

With that, Betty scrunches her fists, tucks them under her double chin like a prissy, gigantic chipmunk and squeaks a petulant "No!" Her mockery, meant only to pique, pierces like sabotage to the heart of me. Tears slide into my eyes. Sobs I cannot strangle sound in my throat. Everyone is looking at me.

"What is it, Mary-Lou?" Her eyes look into mine as if she would read my mind.

"I don't know . . . I don't know . . ." I cry, holding back the knowing that threatens, slouching, from some black hole of loss, some orphan loneliness that is my home. The acoustics of my sorrow sound like screaming in a tunnel.

"Tell," she urges softly, as if I knew. She lifts her hand to my face. I flinch, as if I were expecting a slap. The touch of her fingers, gentle on my cheek, opens the sanctuary where the child takes refuge. "Who are you?" she whispers into the dark.

"Mommy!" I wail, collapsing into Betty's lap. "Mommy, it's not fair." Anger, as old as the rocking chair, finds its voice.

"It's all right," Betty whispers, rubbing my back in soft circles. "It isn't fair, is it?" she asks herself, like a child. "Of course it isn't," she answers in sweet consolation, stroking my hair, kneading my heaving shoulders. "It isn't fair at all."

Little by little, I become aware of the sounds of my own sorrow, of the weight of my own head, of where I am, and how I am, and who. I do not want to lift my face up into my life. I want to hide myself forever, like a motherless child, safe in the comfort of this fragrant, barren lap.

"You don't have to rush. I'll wait," Chipper calls reassuringly to Peter. Chipper Reingold, né Michael Reingold, Jr., sounds very adult for his six years. In a normal burst of childish energy, he has run across the backyard. Now, as if embarrassed by his own joy, he stands, stock-still, midway between the back door and the jungle gym, waiting for Peter to catch up.

Chipper is Peter's only friend now since Geoffrey defected to Andrew down the street. We bought this house because there were so many tricycles parked in the driveways. That's how many kids there were who weren't going to play with Peter. Defected. The neighborhood is a war zone. The sound of children's laughter from other yards invades like a fifth column and poisons like mustard gas. I wonder if I'd make my kid play with the crippled kid down the block, and I know I wouldn't, I'd suggest it maybe once or twice, and then I'd drop it.

We are *hors de combat* in no man's land. Not too many people drop by. Glenda, Chip's mother, is my main daytime friend. She comes like a volunteer, carrying a white flag, from the outside world, wholesome as Ship 'n Shore and Shetland; starched, pleated and plaid, her brown hair bobbed, her smile wet and white as milk. She reaches her long fingers with their clear, shapely nails through the chicken-wire fencing, to touch me in my quarantine. Most of the time she brings Chipper. She is not afraid that we are catching.

Standing together at the kitchen window, we watch Peter moving toward Chip. We watch Peter struggling after his intention, impelling his body to keep up with the runner in his mind. Inside my skin, I feel my own nerves and muscles tense with imagined speed.

"I don't know how you do it, babe," says Glenda, touching my sleeve.

My heart reaches, and falls back. In her very efforts to console, I discover my otherness. Sometimes I'm a leper. Sometimes I'm a prisoner. And sometimes I'm a monarch in exile—tolerated, even protected. I pose no threat to the present regime. In fact, I am exemplary, essential to it in some way. I am what can happen if. I am there-but-for-the-grace-of-You-Know-Who go you-know-who. I am a tragic celebrity.

"I don't know how you do it," Glenda repeats.

"You don't get a choice. You do it because you have to. If it happened to you, you'd do it too. Then you'd know how I do it." A tragic celebrity is humble.

"I'm not so sure," says Glenda, sitting down at the kitchen table. "I'm not so sure I could."

"I am." I am sure she would be better. She *is* better. It's not just her own doing. She is naturally more satisfied, more sufficient than I. I run on empty. She comes from a long line of love. She has it to spare. I am jealous of her love even as she shares it with me. Even as Chipper plays with Pete, I envy her lucky womb.

"Listen, babe," says Glenny, motioning me to sit down. "There's something I want to discuss with you."

"Is something wrong?" Ours is the parodic woman's world of anecdote and recipe. By silent mutual agreement we keep it that way. Small talk. Safe talk.

"No, not wrong. Just important. Mike and I are thinking about making our wills, not that we have any money to give away. But we figured we should have a will, just in case something should happen to both of us—you know—to appoint guardians for the kids.

"My parents are wonderful," she goes on, "they adore the kids, but we think they're too old to bring up three little kids. Mike's got two unmarried brothers, and I'm an only child ... Mike and I had a long talk about all our relatives and friends, and whom we'd most trust our children with, and we agreed. It's you and Larry. You're the best parents we know. We'd like to put your names in our will as our children's guardians, but—"

"We'd be honored," I interrupt.

Glenda lifts up her hand like a traffic cop. "Not so fast. Think about it. Discuss it with Larry. Think about it as if it was going to happen. Imagine having five children. Imagine trying to incorporate someone else's children into your family. Imagine how jealous your own kids would be if you succeeded. Imagine how much less time you'd have for them if you succeeded. Imagine all the trouble, all the caring, all the worry. Not to mention all the money.

"That's what *we* did. We thought about it long and hard. We made absolutely sure that we would want to take care of your children as our own if anything happened to you and Larry."

"But I—"

"It would have to be reciprocal."

In the silence, her kindness lies before me as vast and unexplored as a new world. I stare at the surface of the table and wait until the wood grain stops swimming beneath my gaze. "You're aware, of course, that you and Mike would be getting the better of the deal," I say when I can speak. "We've only got two kids. You've got three."

I have to make the bed on my knees. One of the wooden legs broke early in our marriage, dumping us slippery and silly on the cold wooden floor. We didn't miss a beat.

Now the bed mocks me as I try to get it even, tugging and tucking the top sheet, testing the tension until it is taut. You could bounce a quarter on it. That is my revenge.

I'm getting compulsive about the sheets; how much of a drop on each side, and whether the pillows should go into the cases tag down, zipper up or vice versa. I can't wait for us to get out of bed in the morning so I can make it, as if there were some evidence to cover up. Now I understand women who annoy by emptying ashtrays at the flick of a spent match. They are not getting laid.

I look up from the execution of a perfect top sheet fold-over at my mother, seated in the chair by the hearth, her lizardskin bag perched on her tweed lap, and suspect that she's one too.

"Is this the woman you told me about?" Mother rummages in her purse and holds out a clipping from the *New York Times*. The scent of sugary decadence from an opened pack of Juicy Fruit gum is released from the reptile's jaws. Mother rewards herself with Juicy Fruit, a half stick at a time.

Like José Ferrer playing Toulouse-Lautrec, I waddle toward her outstretched hand on my knees. "Yup. That's Betty all right. Isn't she great-looking?" I scan the article, hoping that it's positive, hoping that the *New York Times* loves Betty Fuller as much as I do, and hoping it will not matter if they don't. They do. Maybe not *as* much, but they do.

I hand the clipping back to mother and head for the bed. There is a letter from Betty Fuller on the bureau. A green ceramic frog with a golden crown, slightly askew, sits on the envelope as if it were a lily pad. Keep kissing the frog, Larry had said, presenting it to me after our first fight. Sooner or later I turn into a prince. "As a matter of fact, we got a letter from Betty today asking us if we might be interested in participating in a four-month training program at Esalen next fall which she'll be leading."

"Harrumph," Mother says. It's a word I've read a lot, but I've never heard anyone actually say it, except Mother. "You're not considering doing it, are you?"

"No—not really."

Mother examines the clipping ostentatiously. "Is she married?"

"No."

"How much does she weigh?"

"Two hundred and eighty pounds," I announce proudly, as if I were a member of the 4-H Club who grew her.

"Some terrific advertisement for mental health," says Mother.

"I'll get going as soon as I finish making the bed." I change the subject. "I really appreciate your being willing to baby-sit this aft. I don't know what I would have done. I promised Paul Good that I'd meet him at the printer's at three, and then it turned out that Glenda had to take Robin to the Little League try-outs." I pinch the edge of the sheet between thumb and index finger and lift it up until it is stretched tautly into a perfect isosceles triangle. I inspect my percale geometry with rueful pride.

"I'm happy to help you out when I can, dear. As long as I'm not doing anything important. Just be sure that you're home no later than five. I'm due at the Mortimer Coles' at seven."

"Sure, Mom."

"Just don't depend on me. I'm not that kind of a grand-mother."

"Sometimes I'm not that kind of a mother," I answer, but she let's it go. I stand up and fold the white chenille bed-spread back, arrange the pillows side by side so that their bottoms overlap where the spread is folded and their tops touch the headboard. Side by side. His and hers. Nice. Then I grasp the edge of the bedspread and lift it gingerly, cere-moniously, over the plump pillows, as if I have just pro-nounced them dead.

"Why don't you get yourself a maid one day a week, dear? Larry's doing well enough for you to afford one, isn't he? Between the house, your husband, the children—Peter, in particular—and now starting a newspaper, you're spread pa-ritty thin, my daughter. You should get some help."

"You mean a *shvartzeh*?" I tease. "I can't do it. I once tried having a maid, but it didn't work out. I couldn't stop myself from cleaning the house thoroughly for her arrival. I did windows, baseboards—I even washed the kitchen floor—on my knees, of course. Oh the burdens of being a bullshit lib-eral!

"Seriously, Mother, how can I employ a black woman to clean my house while I go to work with Paul Good on *The Turtle* so that maybe we can convince the Westport Board of Education to allow the black kids of the woman from Bridgeport who's cleaning my house to attend the Westport schools so that my kids, when they get to be my age, maybe won't be prejudiced against blacks—like I am."

"You're not prejudiced against blacks, dear. You've

disrupted your whole life to work on that newspaper. Look what you're doing for them. You deserve one."

Mother, a sly smile spreading on her face, her thumbs pressed flat and white against the shiny mahogany surface, begins to sink slowly, silently beneath the dining-room table. Her strained expression contorts into panic. Mother is in trouble. We hear muffled, thumping noises. She is flailing madly with her legs. She cannot find the buzzer. Suddenly her face registers success, and then snooty tranquillity. Right on cue, Eddie Mae Borges and a leg of lamb rampant elbow their way through the swinging kitchen door, which snaps menacingly at her heels.

Eddie Mae Borges is the new shvartzeh *who is "working out quite well," as far as Mother is concerned. Mother jokes about Eddie Mae's newly acquired married name, which is Portuguese. This, Mother explains, is a "step up" for Eddie Mae on the racial rungs of the color ladder, making of Eddie Mae "a higher type of* shvartzeh *than your usual," although her elevated social position creates its own problems. Eddie Mae has recently served notice that she will no longer get down on her hands and knees and wash the kitchen floor.*

"How do you like them apples!" Mother asks, her voice strident with rhetorical idiom. "Actually," she adds more soberly, "only Hungarian girls are willing to get down on their hands and knees and scrub anymore. The Irish might still do it, but then you're lucky if they don't steal, or drink, or both."

"What's Paul Good's background?" Mother asks. She means is he Jewish.

"He's a freelance writer. He writes for *Life* and lots of other magazines. The *Times,* even. He's written a lot about blacks and injustice. Long before this local issue came up. It's his devotion." I see Paul on a white charger, tilting at life. "Sir Freelance A Lot."

Mother doesn't laugh; she is intent upon tracking the

scent. "Do you know anything else about his background, dear?"

"You mean like if he's got all his shots?" I'll be grown up, I figure, when I stop making this so hard for her.

" 'Good' sounds like a Jewish name."

"Ahhhhhh," I exclaim in a declining arc, "you mean is Paul Good Jewish?"

"Yes," Mother admits.

"No, he's not." I am as perversely pleased about Paul Good's Catholicism as I am about Betty Fuller's outlandish size. "He's an Irish Catholic."

"Does he drink?" Mother asks.

Mother is the Margaret Mead of bigots.

"How were things at the office today," I ask automatically and then recoil with chagrin when I realize that I sound like a wife. "Jeezus!" I scold myself out loud while dishing out the macaroni and cheese. "There's one I swore I'd never say, along with 'Hot enough for you?' "

"Don't ask," Larry moans. "And there's one *I* swore I'd never say."

"We got our report cards today," says Adam, talking with his mouth full.

"Don't talk with your mouth full, dear, it's not polite." The words are out before I remember that I once promised myself—the way I promised myself so often as a child that I would always remember a certain place or a certain moment, forever—that I would never, ever talk like a parent. I would never say "Now run along and play" or "When you get a little older, you'll thank me" or "This hurts me more than it hurts you," or my all-time personal favorite, "That's very good, dear, what did Ronnie get?"

"I got an A in English, and an A in social studies, and an A in math," Adam announces, and I hate myself so much for wondering if anyone got an A-plus that I don't ask.

"That's terrific," says Larry, putting down his fork to

shake Adam's waiting hand. "I'm really proud of you. Aren't you, Mom?"

My fourth-grade social studies teacher, Miss Falkowski, is getting annoyed with the class. "Why," she says, sending an exasperated whoosh of air through her nostrils, "must I always see the same hands?"

"Oh, Miss Falkowski, I know, I know, I know, oh please, Miss Falkowski, I know, I know, oh please, please, teacher, please, teacher, call on me!" I hiss and gasp, flinging my body across the top of my desk. Straining forward ever more obliquely, my left hand is propped on its elbow, throwing me off balance, holding aloft my waving right arm. I have to stick one foot out into the aisle to serve as a flying buttress.

"Come on, class," says Miss Falkowski, her hands on her hips, her toes tapping, her hawk eyes surveying the classroom. "I want to see some new hands."

Yearning, fervent, I pray that no new hands will go up. "Oh please, God, oh please, God, oh please, God." They don't.

Miss Falkowski's voice is heavy and ironic with mock defeat. "Yes, Mary-Lou?" she sighs as her index finger dips through the air in my direction.

"Anthracite and bituminous," I answer, breathless from the sudden release of so much impatient ardor.

"You are a suck and a brown nose" reads the note that Jimmy Petrantonio drops on my lap on his way to the boys' room.

"And an A in Follow Directions and Works Easily with Others," Adam brags on. "I'm a genius."

"That *is* terrific." I smile, leaning over to kiss him on the nose. "You are a genius. But even if you got awful marks, I'd still love you just as much," I add, never forgetting Peter.

"What's an A?" Peter asks.

"It's the best mark you can get at school," I answer. "You

don't get marks yet because you're in kindergarten, but when you're in the first grade you'll get marks too."

"Will I want them?" Peter asks.

Peter does not yet work easily with concepts, judging size relationships, or counting, and his progress in the pre-reading group has been slight. He is easily frustrated and becomes angry with himself and others quite often. It is our feeling that Peter's needs may be better met in a two-year kindergarten program at Bayberry, rather than by placement in the first grade,

reads Pete's report card which arrived today and lies on the kitchen counter, reinserted in its envelope.

"Sure you'll want them," says Adam, who has decided to take over the explanation. "Marks tell how you're doing in school. Everybody wants to get A's. That's the best you can do. There's A's and B's and C's and D's. A is best; then comes B, that's good; and then comes C and that's just fair; and then comes D. That's doo-doo."

"Well, what do you do with the marks when you get them?" Pete asks, reaching over his plate, two-fisted, for his milk.

"You just *get* them, and then you *have* them. They mean you're smart, that you're a genius at doing things, like I am," Adam declares in a high-bouncing balloon of a boast. Suddenly I hate him.

"Grades aren't that important, Adam," I interrupt, as if I am no longer the same sweaty mother whose intellectual blood lust, just moments ago, drove her to distraction over A-pluses. His happy face flinches and shatters as he senses my treachery.

"It's more important how kind you are, and how honest, and loving," I go on, until I notice Larry looking down a slightly wrinkled nose at me as if something smells bad, like bullshit.

Then I realize that what I really mean is that grades must not be important because Petie still holds up four fingers when he means that he is five, and that it is more important to be kind because Petie still tries to nail the square blocks in the round hole in the wooden post office on Dr. Braverman's play table. And I mean it is also important to be honest because Petie will never be smart enough or live long enough to go to college, anyway, so how could grades be important? And I stress how important it is to be a loving person because Pete's life cannot be measured in expectations and accomplishments. Somehow—but oh my God I cannot imagine how—Peter's life must grow steadily and bravely upward, against a declining graph line of utter failure. On this graph, each day, blocked off like a cell, is a new low. Each day charts new insults and deprivations, all that the unrelenting body can visit upon itself, all with excruciating attention paid to detail: the day the scissors feel stiff in his hand; the day the pedals won't turn on the bike; the day his knees buckle; the day he cannot raise his hand to get called on in school; the day the fork falls from his fingers. Each day, until everything, all, has been taken, extracted from him— the last step taken, the last breath drawn, until, finally, the line on the graph above his hospital bed slouches and goes flat.

I look to Pete and try to read the expression on his face. He seems neither injured by Adam's boast nor cognizant of my efforts to assuage his presumed pain.

"You're right, Adam," says Pete, carrying the glass back across his plate and setting it down, the tip of his tongue a dot of milky pink determination receding into his mouth. "You *are* a genius at doing, but are you a genius at just plain being?" Pete speaks in a tone which I am expecting to be taunting, playground-snide. But it isn't. His voice is as innocent, wise and penetrating as a prophet's.

Milk spills, chairs scrape away from the table, and Peter is falling through the air backwards, toward the brick kitchen floor, his eyes wide and staring, his mouth open. He lands. Frozen in a spasm of breathlessness, his lips compressed bluish white against his teeth, Peter waits to be able to cry. I cannot move.

"He just fell over! He just fell over, Mommy!" cries Adam, and my heart bleeds for him. But when I try to say, "It's okay, Adam. I can't blame you for hating him sometimes," I find I am unable to speak. I am holding my breath with Peter.

"You just can't do that, no matter how angry you feel," Larry is saying with great tenderness, encouraging a reluctant Adam to approach. When his arm rests around Adam's shoulders and he feels Adam's body relax against his own, Larry goes on. "No matter how much you want to hit Pete, you just must not do it. You have to stop yourself. You have an unfair advantage. Peter is younger, and smaller, and his balance isn't as good as yours. When you push him over on the hard floor, you hurt him too much. I can't let you do that. You'll have to start finding some other way to be angry with your brother," he finishes, giving Adam a little satisfied squeeze. "Now get lost. Botha youze guys. Yeah, you too, squirt," he adds, picking up a sniffling Pete and setting him gently down on his feet. "Beat it!"

Pete lumbers after Adam down the hall, touching the walls for balance.

"Peter is beginning to fall down a lot," I say to Larry when I'm sure the children will not overhear. I cannot bring myself to look at him. I am so ashamed, so disappointed in myself. In almost three years of trying I have not, so far, been able to cure Peter.

"I know," says Larry, looking into his hands. "I've noticed." His shoulders seem slack and weighted.

Oh, Larry! Don't give up, don't give up! I'm working on a cure. So far it hasn't succeeded, but it's still early. Three years isn't a long time for an incurable disease. I just need more time. I want to explain, except that if I did, I would have to hear myself say that I graze my lips lightly, lovingly, surreptitiously against the knees of Pete's corduroy overalls as I take his clothes from the bureau each morning to bless them, and that at bedtime I kiss the enlarged calf on each leg, where muscle is being turned into fat and the disease's grim manufacture is already evident. I would have to hear myself say that each night before I go to sleep I conspire with God, or with Satan—which one is my religion I am not sure—and together we conjure up an image of Peter running.

It helps to start by imagining his hair like fluid poured, caught in a photographic, midair moment, perpetually spilling, bouncing on air. Once his hair is set in motion I work on his reluctant body, picturing a forward thrusting of the shoulders, and a pumping of the arms that is not so grim and determined as Peter's really is but, instead, smooth and loose. And finally the legs. Instead of working them up and down in place, like Br'er Rabbit struggling with the Tar Baby, I make Pete's legs reach through the air in great strides, exercising them until they move with the idealized gait of a champion horse I remember from a film clip, frolicking in slow-motion glory, defining equipoise. I am wishing him well.

If I tell Larry about these secret rites, then both of us will think that I am crazy.

"Do you think we should have chosen the heel-cord operation for Peter?" I say instead.

"No," Larry answers. "I think we were right to follow our instincts on that one. I don't regret the decision. I'm just scared about what we have to face, what Peter has to face. I'm worried about me, I'm worried about you, and I'm worried about Adam, especially. This could be toughest on him."

"Mommy, Muh-ommy!" we hear Peter shrieking from the other end of the house. "Mommy! Mommy! Mommy!" accelerates our pace down to the end of the hall where Larry and I scramble with all four hands to find the knob and push open our bedroom door.

Adam is standing in the middle of the bed, holding a dangling Peter upright by the front of his shirt, attempting to stand him up on his feet again, however briefly, so that he may push him over again.

All three of us watch Peter begin to lose his balance, tip over and fall, gently, irredeemably backwards through the air, and land softly on target, a heap of cumulus pillows with which Adam has scrupulously banked the wooden head-board.

"Bombs away!" Adam proclaims.

"Hot off the press, ladies and gentlemen! Extra! Extra!" Larry Palaia of the Remar Press delivers the first copy of *The Turtle* from the whirling, clattering machinery and holds it up like a newborn. Then he brings it over to Paul and me.

"It's beautiful." I run my fingers along the soft, smooth surface, celebrating it tangibly. "Don't you think so, Paul?"

Paul reaches for the paper. I watch the muscle strands play themselves beneath the skin of his forearm, like the keys on a player piano. While he studies the front page, I study him—blue eyes under heavy lids; nose somewhat asymmetrically located, pushed there no doubt in a street fight. His medium-sized sturdy build—the flat belly showing the middle-aged man's will not to go soft—bristles with contentious energy.

" 'Behold the turtle,' " he reads, " 'he maketh progress by sticking his neck out.' Yeah, I like it . . . Looks good. The boldface looks good." Each word is a concession. He talks out of one side of his mouth like Nathan Detroit and handles his cigar like Groucho Marx.

"Hey," says Larry Palaia, "where did you guys get that saying—from some President or something?"

"I don't know who said it first, but I first heard it from a friend of mine, Bill Gailmor," I answer. "He was a journalist and radio news commentator in the forties, before he was blacklisted. He died last year of a brain tumor. Bill had a collection of miniature turtles. His wife gave me one. It was carved from white onyx."

I saw Bill in his hospital room. He was sitting up in bed, smiling, nodding, thanking me for a book he would never read. I put it on top of the stack of books on his bedside table, the spines of which read like the latest "Editor's Choice" list in the *New York Times Book Review*. Like the ancient Egyptians, all his friends must have believed that Bill would need his books in the next life, even though he could no longer read them in this.

"The boldface definitely looks sharper than the small caps." Paul opens the paper and lays it down on one of the long, narrow oak tables that divide the huge workroom into columns. Decades of inky fingers handling thousands of pieces of type have dyed the wood grain black.

Boldface. Small caps. Bodoni. Flush left. Logo. Blue pencil. I love the lingo! I love it the way some women thrill to their lover's passionate, pornographic entreaties during intercourse. I would get it on with Quasimodo if he showed me his press card.

"I'll give you guys a few minutes to gloat, and then we'll start the run." Palaia grins a boyish grin. "Don't worry. I won't charge you time and a half."

Paul and I laugh; he isn't charging us at all. "I don't like the way they're treating those kids from Bridgeport. It ain't right" was the reason he offered to print our newspaper free.

"The logo looks good," I remark to Paul. "Hey! Don't turn the page so fast! I want to savor it!"

It's true, the logo does look good, but what I really want to savor is the name my greedy eyes just caught a glimpse of. Mine. My by-line. Me. My eyes can't get enough. They want to read and reread each tiny, sturdy little cap and lower case. My ego wants to bounce up and down on that tough little hyphen as if it were a trampoline. But he turns the page, anyway.

"How does my editorial look to you?"

"It's great."

"You really think so?" Paul looks skeptical.

"This is the best part." I take the paper away from him and read: " 'The silent ones, we believe, are a minority, not a majority. But they are numerous. They are the commuters who ride past Harlem each day and—if they are moved to think at all—wonder why blacks don't do something to improve themselves. They make no connections between the absence of black faces on the commuter trains, and the segregated lives at 125th Street. They know that in the business world, doors open on doors through personal contact, mutual experiences and all the other ruboffs from white middle-class life style. Yet they would deny black children the chance their fathers didn't have to "learn" the society that presently controls their destinies. They would break a man's leg and condemn him because he limps.' "

"I hope we're not just talking to ourselves," says Paul, thrusting his hands into his pockets.

"Of course we're not. The *Westport News* has been slanting the news about Project Concern for weeks now. It's the only source of information the people in town have had. Now that *The Turtle*'s on the scene, people are going to change their minds; I know it." I hear in my voice the same heady mix of spanielly devotion and Bryn Mawr lust that Katharine Hepburn felt for Spencer Tracy. "What about 'and the truth shall set them free'? What about *that*?"

"Bigots don't get set free. Bigots don't change their minds. Out here in the two-acre greenswards of what the newspapers like to call 'affluent Fairfield County,' it's hard to tell a bigot. They don't say 'nigger.' In fact, they go to no end of fancy verbal footwork to let you know that they're not bigots. Quite the contrary. They're *humanitarians*. They're going to vote against Project Concern because they're worried that the poor, impressionable little black kids will get depressed when they have to get bused back to their ghettos after spending the school day enjoying our middle-class goodies. As if the kids hadn't seen all those luxuries on TV programs and commercials since they were born. They probably even manage to convince themselves that they're humanitarians, but they don't convince me. They're bigots and they'll stay bigots no matter what information we offer."

"So what's the point? What are we breaking our asses for?"

"Maybe, just maybe," he concedes, "we can win some converts among those people who have gotten caught in the cross-fire between the bigots and the good guys. But that's the most we can hope for, and they may not be enough to swing the vote," he cautions.

"I didn't think the situation was that grim."

"Hey, kid, when you've been at this as long as I have, you get used to losing. Besides"—he reaches into his back pocket for his billfold—"losing isn't the worst thing that can happen to you." Paul removes a tiny square of folded paper and hands it to me. "Take a look at that."

The paper, thin and soft in my hands, opens almost automatically along folds soiled and frayed by use. I begin to read.

One of the Just Men came to Sodom, determined to save the inhabitants from sin and punishment. Night and day he walked the streets and markets preaching against greed and theft, falsehood and indifference. In the beginning people listened and smiled ironically. Then they stopped listening; he no longer even amused them. Killers went on killing, the wise kept silent, as if there was no Just Man in their midst.

One day a child, moved by compassion for the unfortunate stranger-preacher, approached him with these words: "Poor stranger, you shout and expend yourself body and soul. Don't you see that it is hopeless?"

"Yes, I see," answered the Just Man.

"Then why do you go on?"

"I'll tell you why. In the beginning, I thought I could change man. Today I know I cannot. If I still shout today, if I still scream, it is to prevent man from ultimately changing me."

"Where's that from?" I ask, looking up from the paper.

"The Talmud. Let me take a look at the rest. I want to make sure they spelled my name right." Paul picks up the paper and scans the pages from top to bottom. "Hey, hey, hey! I didn't see this one before. 'Bill Gailmor—The Man Behind the Motto.' Where'd it come from?"

"I wrote it at the last minute. The cartoon we were counting on didn't get here in time, so I filled in the hole."

Paul reads silently, intently.

"You weren't here. I had to."

Paul begins to read aloud. " 'When Bill wrote a column for the New York *Daily Compass,* he established the Exalted and Independent Order of the Turtle and invited his readers to nominate Americans they thought most deserving of the honor, courageous people who had stuck their necks out in the face of dire peril. Bill, as he himself would have said, was enturtled to the title as much as anyone . . .' 'Enturtled to the title'?" Paul repeats, throwing his head back to laugh. "I like that. Y'know, kid, for a housewife, you're not a bad writer."

"Where are we goin' in the car?" Pete finally asks after handing the quarter to the toll collector. "Uh-oh!" he adds darkly. "I think I gave my lolly to the tollhouse-cookie man."

"The poor bastard probably can't get his hand open," says Larry.

"Where are we going?" Pete asks again.

"Quack," quacks Larry.

"Are we goin' to Zinzyland? Are we gonna see Donald Duck?"

"No, sweetie. Daddy's only fooling. We're going to see a man."

"What kind of a man?" Pete asks.

"Quack!"

"A nice man."

"What kind of a nice man, Mommy?"

"Quack!"

"You're not much of a duck," I offer.

"You're not much of a liar," Larry responds.

What the hell am I supposed to tell him? You see, Pete, your crazy parents are taking you to a healer. Mommy met this nice lady named Joyce Goodrich, Ph.D., who told her about this nice man named Lawrence LeShan, Ph.D., who believes that by entering into an altered state of consciousness, some people can heal others. LeShan was chief of the research project on the paranormal at the New York State Psychiatric Research Center. He has a grant from the McDonnell Foundation to investigate healers and healing. It's words like "research project," "grant" and "Ph.D." that get your mommy every time.

Eat me. Drink me. Swallow me whole. I go Alice one better as I slip right out of my mind, down the rabbit hole and through the looking glass. What can I tell you, Pete? It could be off with our heads.

"But *where* are we going?" Pete insists.

"Lourdes," says Larry.

"We're going to New York. Let's see which one of us sees the Empire State Building first."

"But *why* am I going to New York?" Pete implores.

"To see a man," I answer.

"Run. See Jane run," Larry mutters.

"But why does he want to see me?" Pete asks.

"Because he likes little boys," I answer, cringing at my own idiocy.

"See Dick run. See Mom sweat," Larry says to the rearview mirror.

"Why isn't Adam coming? Doesn't the man want to see Adam, too?"

"Adam's bigger than you. This man likes little boys especially."

"Now she's in big trouble, Spot," says Larry to the mirror.

"Does Adam know I am going to New York with you? Does Adam know? Does he, Mommy? Does he?" Pete asks intently.

"Of course, darling, he knows. He's at Glenda's house.

We'll pick him up on the way back from New York." I reach for Peter, who is standing on the seat between us, looking out the rear window, and draw him down on my lap. "You're a Snerdly Bumpforth and I love you," I say into the nape of his neck.

"Kisses are bad for you," says Pete. "You put your lips on the back of my neck and the germs from your kisses leak through my skin, and they meet my germs, and my germs and your germs fight, and my germs lose, and I get sick. But keep on doing it anyway, it feels so good."

"I love you, Pete" is all I can say.

"Does Glenda know I'm going to New York?"

"I suppose so. I suppose I told her we were going to New York when I brought Adam over. Why do you ask? Why do you want to know, you little question monster? That's what I'm going to call you from now on. Mommy's little freckle-faced question monster."

"Does Robin know? Does Chipper know?"

"Know what, darling?"

"Know I'm here," Pete answers slowly, vaguely, as if for a moment he has forgotten the question, right in the middle of answering it.

"Mommy, is it true what Freddie says?"

"What does Freddie say, darling?"

"Is it true that I'm going to be in a wheelchair soon?"

I tighten my arms around him and draw him toward me, the way a harpist embraces her harp, my hands pressing against his ribs to quiet his trembling and mine.

"Yes. Shoo-shoo, baby, shoo-shoo-shoo," we rock in time with the white-music sound of tires on macadam at sixty miles an hour. Chanting, I stare over Peter's head and through the windshield as if I believe that like the broken white lines, we can be sucked to oblivion beneath the car.

Then I hear myself speaking. "Petie, shall I tell you why? I think it is time. Before you know it, you'll be six. I think you are old enough, a big enough boy to know. Do you want to know?"

Peter does not answer.

"Sweetie, you have a muscle problem. Your muscles are getting weaker, and when they get too weak to help you walk around, then you'll need a wheelchair. The disease you have has a name. It's called muscular dystrophy. That's why it is so hard for you to run."

"That's bad," says Peter, who does not have a vocabulary for sorrow.

Oh, save us, save us, Larry, I cry within. We are lost!

"It's not *so* bad," says Larry, taking his right hand off the wheel to touch Peter's knee. I am so grateful that Larry can speak. "You probably don't know this, Pete, but one of the finest Presidents the United States ever had was in a wheelchair. Did you ever hear of Franklin Delano Roosevelt?"

"No," says Pete.

"Well," Larry continues, gathering momentum, arguing the case for paraplegia, "ol' Franklin Delano managed to become one of the most important men of his time even though he was in a wheelchair. It'll be tough, Pete"—Larry's voice softens—"it'll definitely be tough, but Mommy and Adam and I will always be here to help you when you need help. That's a promise."

I watch Larry fighting for our life. This is the toughest case he's ever tried. A real loser.

"It's bad," Peter repeats.

"I can think of a lot worse things than being in a wheelchair." Undaunted, Larry carries on.

"I can't," says Peter in a tone that I have never heard—flat, airless, adult.

"For instance," says Larry, pausing for just a moment, "I think it would be worse to be blind. After all, even if you can't walk because of a muscle problem, you can still get to any place you want to go in a wheelchair or in a car. And you don't even have to push. There are motorized wheelchairs that you can drive all by yourself."

"Do they go fast?" Pete asks.

"Pretty darn fast," says Larry, "and you don't even get tired. But if you can't see, there is nothing you can do instead of seeing. You wouldn't even be able to see Mommy's face, or my face . . ."

"Or Adam's face," Pete joins in, cautiously.

"Or even your own silly face," Larry says tenderly, "although maybe that wouldn't be such a bad idea, since you're soooo funny-looking."

"I guess you're right," Pete concludes. "Look-it, Daddy, look-it, Mommy! The Umpire Scrape Building!"

"LeShan, LeShan, LeShan . . ." I bump my finger down the row of embossed plastic names alongside the row of doorbells in the lobby of the brownstone on Seventy-fifth Street. "What kind of name is LeShan?" The moment the words escape my lips, I want to disown them.

"You sound like your mother," Larry comments.

I nod miserably. "At least give me credit for not saying"—and here I draw myself up to my haughtiest—"It shaure ain't Fa-rench." Then I drop my voice to a conspiratorial hush and deliver the coup de grâce of whispered maternal pronunciamentos, "It's been *changed.*"

"Changed" is one of the six words so awful that Mother will only whisper them loudly. The others are "nose job," "cancer," "homosexual," *"shvartzeh"* and "Jewish."

"LeShan, LeShan . . . here it is." I poise my finger on the button and look up at Larry. "Ready?"

He nods. "Just for the record, though, let it be known that next to marrying you, this is the craziest thing I've ever done."

"Duly noted." I press the buzzer. "We'll both plead insanity."

"Temporary, I trust."

"Pick me, pick me, pick me like a grape," says Petie, reaching toward Larry, opening and closing his fingers.

"Consider yourself picked." He bends over to lift Pete in his arms.

I wait with my hand on the knob for the corresponding buzz. It has begun. We are embarked on a trip down our very own Yellow Brick Road. So what, then, have I come for—courage? a heart? Or maybe just a ticket, sir, please, sir, a one-way ticket back to Kansas, back to before the tornado hit.

The buzzer sounds, splicing my nerves. I turn the knob and open the door. We step through to find ourselves in yet another lobby. This one has two doors.

"I feel like the guy in 'The Lady or the Tiger,' " Larry whispers.

"I'm Dorothy in Oz."

"In that case," says Larry, "I must be the Scarecrow."

"What did *he* want? I forget."

"A brain" is all he has time to say before the door on the right opens and the space in the dimly lit doorway is authoritatively filled by a very tall, robust middle-aged man dressed in an open-necked shirt, tan trousers and worn black leather slippers.

"Come in, come in." He steps back from the door to allow us to enter. "I bet you're hot and tired after that long drive," he addresses Peter. "Would you like to rest?"

Peter, who hardly ever wants to rest, says yes.

"There's a sofa in this back room." LeShan indicates the room to the left. He leads the way and Larry follows, with Pete in his arms. "And, Mrs. Weisman, why don't you just go take a seat in my office." He nods with his head toward the room on the right.

"So . . ." says LeShan when he and Larry have joined me in the office. "Tell me how I can help you."

We seem to be at a loss for words.

"Come, come, you must be here for something." He picks up his pipe from the desk, lights it, leans back in his chair and punctuates the air with little explosive puffs. This man is a fake. I can tell. People with real Ph.D.s don't come in this size. And they don't parody themselves with pipe and slippers. LeShan, my ass. LeSham is more like it.

"Come, come!" He smiles encouragingly.

I cannot bring myself to say, "We're here for you to cure Peter." That is just too crazy.

"It's not every day"—LeShan breaks the silence—"that you find yourself talking to a mad scientist who experiments with the paranormal. Actually, I'm rather overrated. People tend to hype that sort of thing."

"Are you saying, then, that you can't help our son?" Larry cross-examines.

"Oh dear," says LeShan, furrowing his face into an expression of consternation behind a puff of smoke, "I'm sure Joyce Goodrich didn't say I could heal your son. I'm a research psychologist, not a mystic. I wish I could heal your son, but I can't. It is possible, though, that he could heal himself."

"I don't understand. Would you please clarify that?" Larry prosecutes.

"I'll do my best, but a little willing suspension of disbelief on your part would be helpful." LeShan leans back, sinks his huge frame even deeper into the leather chair and smiles. Smoke leaks out of his mouth and floats upward, momentarily obscuring his features.

"In the course of studying and testing various well-known healers throughout the world, I have developed a theory that I'm currently involved in testing." LeShan sucks deeply and shoots the smoke out one corner of his mouth.

"No psychic healer does very well. Twenty percent success on a good day is hot stuff. The one exception was born in Bethlehem a long time ago, and you've got to remember"—LeShan admonishes by wagging the stem of his pipe at us—"He had a very good press. We don't know about His failures, if any.

"Most alleged cases of healing, when closely examined, turn out to be due to suggestion. There are, however, half a dozen or so healers whose work has consistently held up under carefully controlled laboratory investigations. We've done blind studies and double blind studies. Psychic healing is a real phenomenon. It's a fact—an impossible fact for some, a threatening fact to others, and, to some members of the scientific community, a fact which must be reckoned with.

"In the course of interviewing these psychic healers, I found them to be curiously ignorant about how they actually heal people. Many claim that they are merely a channel through which God works; one guy said he was effective only when he lined himself up with the meridians of the earth's magnetic field, north and south. He showed me how he did it. He was lined up east and west!" LeShan chuckles, clenching his pipe in his teeth. "The most intelligent psychics say they don't know how they do it.

"But they all agree on a couple of points. Each talks about uniting with the healee's own innate capacity to heal himself, and they all agree that in order for healing to take place one must experience a shift in consciousness."

"Bullshit" is what I feel like yelling, but I don't. Instead I just throw a verbal flag on the play, a fifteen-yard penalty for fuzzy thinking. "I don't even know what you mean by 'shift in consciousness,'" I protest.

"I know you don't," LeShan answers, "but it has a real meaning nevertheless. People have more or less resistance to unification. Trying to unite with some people is like throwing a rubber ball against a brick wall in the hope that it will stick." LeShan pauses for a few seconds while I get the point. "Sometimes it works. Sometimes it doesn't. The healer changes the metaphysical system, and the healee sometimes responds."

"Hardly an exact science," I mutter.

"Hardly," LeShan agrees amiably. "There's a gentleman who lives in England by the name of Chapman-Lang who has a particularly good record as a healer. You might consider making an appointment to take Peter to see him. He lives in a small town—Aylesbury—outside London."

"Is he a doctor?"

"No," LeShan answers with a hint of a smile. "He's not even a Ph.D. He's a member of the Aylesbury Fire Brigade. Or at least he's a part-time fireman.

"A few years ago George Chapman discovered, quite suddenly and much to his surprise, that he could go into a trance state and become the medium for a William Lang, an ophthalmic surgeon who died many years before, in 1937, I believe. Mr. Lang had been a highly respected surgeon in his day; he published many scholarly papers in the medical journals, and in addition to his appointment to the Middlesex Hospital in 1880, served as a consultant specialist at a number of well-known London hospitals. Apparently none of his contemporaries found him weird. He is described as a cultured, dignified, well-connected man, a favorite of the Duke and Duchess of Bedford. Lang had a reputation for kindness.

"Chapman the fireman apparently goes into a trance and becomes the deceased Mr. Lang. He not only speaks like him, Chapman's working-class accent being replaced by Lang's upper-class diction, but he seems to grow older and hunched, like the elderly Mr. Lang.

"If Lang was a doctor," Larry interrups, "why do you call him 'mister'?"

"In England it's the custom to call a doctor with a mastership in surgery by that title."

"I never knew that," says Larry. "Forgive me for interrupting. Please continue."

"In the trance state, but only in the trance state, Chapman is able to diagnose diseases, recognize and share medical information with Lang's former students, now middle-aged practicing physicians themselves, and to effect remarkable cures on patients whom the traditional medical community has pronounced 'hopeless.'

"Chapman was just a small boy when Lang died. He hadn't known him. And up until Chapman was somehow elected to be the medium for the deceased Lang, he had no medical knowledge at all. He has been a garage hand and a butcher, and served with the RAF during the war. Even so, only Chapman in trance has medical knowledge, not Chapman in his normal frame of mind.

"Mr. Lang had a son—Basil, I think his name was—who was also a surgeon, and who predeceased his father. Basil is known to assist Chapman-Lang during operations."

"Operations? What operations?" I cry.

LeShan laughs. "Chapman-Lang operates on what people call the spirit body. Other people call it the aura. It's a concept I've never really understood, although some reputable people seem to."

"You don't believe all this, do you?" Larry asks, incredulous.

"I'm a scientist, not a spiritualist, and I'm certainly not Chapman-Lang's advocate. I am merely telling you that he appears to assume this deceased doctor's identity and medical skills, and that he does have to his credit a number of verifiable cures."

"What does he charge?"

"I believe he charges about two pounds. Not enough to get rich on. I mentioned him only to be helpful. If the prospect disturbs you, please forget it."

"I can't forget it now," I mutter. "It's like the peacock's eye."

"Peacock's eye?" asks LeShan.

"Mary-Lou means the fairy tale about a man who hears about a witch who can turn anything into gold. Naturally the man is eager to learn the secret, so he goes to visit the witch, ready to extract the secret from her by any means. Instead, the witch surprises him by readily agreeing to tell him the magical incantation. 'It's that simple?' the man says, unable to believe his good fortune. 'Yes,' the old crone replies, 'except for one thing. Each time, before you recite the incantation I have just taught you, you must be sure never, ever to think of a peacock's eye.' "

"I see." LeShan rocks slightly in his chair. "I appreciate

your problem. Perhaps I can help you to extricate yourselves with a little demonstration of my own. As I said earlier, one of the prime requisites for healing is the capacity to shift your state of consciousness. I have trained myself to do this. In fact, my hypothesis is that everyone has this innate capacity, to a greater or lesser extent. With your permission, I will try to demonstrate this now with your son."

"I appreciate the offer," I say, "but, quite frankly, I don't want to upset Peter." What I really mean is, this charade has gone far enough.

"You have nothing to lose, Mrs. Weisman. He's resting in the other room."

I look to Larry, who shrugs his approval.

Hope and cynicism are performing isometrics in my brain.

"I'm afraid you're going to be rather disappointed. There are no incantations, no hocus-pocus, no thunderclaps or bolts of lightning. I'm just going to close my eyes. It helps me to concentrate."

"Is there anything we should do or not do?" I ask. "Should we close our eyes too?" I do not like to be left out of anything.

"No. You and Mr. Weisman just sit there quietly." LeShan rolls up his shirt sleeves. "It's hot in here, even with the air conditioning," he says, adding with a smile in our direction, "although I don't suppose it's quite so hot for the skeptical."

LeShan closes his eyes, rests his elbow on his right knee and his forehead in the splay stretching between thumb and first finger.

Larry and I exchange rolled-up whites-of-the-eyes glances, don't-ask-me shoulder shrugs, and concentric, spiral circlings of the index finger at the temple, until we run out of pantomimes of mockery.

When at last, after about ten minutes, LeShan raises his head, we have both folded our hands in our laps, like schoolchildren who've been passing notes while the teacher was writing on the blackboard.

"Peter and I united easily," he reports with a smile. "I met virtually no resistance. He's very available, very open and unguarded. I had no trouble at all contacting him. He's a very special child, although I expect you must know that better than I." LeShan looks at us with a new intimacy and without a trace of his former humor.

"I sensed a secure, happy and beloved child. I tried to convey that feeling to him, and Peter seemed to communicate back to me the five-year-old's equivalent of 'So what else is new?' "

"That's very nice," I say as sweetly as possible, when what I really am is angry and desperate to get away from this crazy fraud and go be ashamed of myself in private. "I'll get Peter," I say, standing up and moving toward the door. LeShan stands too.

"Come on! Get up! Time to go home now!" I call peremptorily to Pete, who is lying down on the sofa.

"I don't want to go home yet, Mommy," he protests from my arms as I carry him down the hall and back into LeShan's office. "It's my turn. Now it's my turn to play." I set him down carefully on the floor. As I reach for my purse, preparing to leave, Pete walks sway-backed and on tiptoe over to LeShan's chair and sits down.

"Now," Pete says to LeShan, "please come over and sit on my lap."

I am about to protest, but LeShan raises both hands, palms up, in front of his chest in a gesture of affectionate surrender to Peter, and then, smiling, hovers gingerly, weightlessly, just a fraction of an inch above Peter's lap.

"Now *this* time," Petie chirps happily at LeShan, "I'll be the ventriloquist, and *you* be the dummy."

Look up. Looggup. Looggup. Loog gup at me. Loog gup at me. Loog gup pat me. Loog gup pat me. I am sitting up in bed, shoulder to shoulder with Larry. He is reading. I am concentrating on him like a child or a witch, attempting to mesmerize him with my will. Loog gup pat me.

He is reading his college paperback copy of George Eliot's *Middlemarch* for the fourth time. After ten years, the inelastic binding glue is cracking and breaking up, and little opaque, amber crumbs lie scattered on the sheets. Loog gup pat me.

"I can't stop thinking about what happened in LeShan's office this afternoon," I finally say aloud.

"What do you mean 'what happened in LeShan's office this afternoon'?" Larry closes *Middlemarch* with a slap and looks up.

"Come on, Larry, you know. Something extraordinary went on between Peter and LeShan. You must have noticed. I mean, can you think of a better description of what extra-sensory perception must be like, especially for a five-year-old, than the metaphor of ventriloquist and dummy?"

"It occurred to me," says Larry, collecting the crumbs one by one between his thumb and forefinger, and depositing them in the palm of his left hand.

"Oh! So it *occurred* to you, did it?"

"You're carping, Mary-Lou. For Chrissakes, stop carping. I give up. You win. I'll talk about it," he grimaces in surrender. "It also occurred to me that there is another possible interpretation of what happened today. It might have been a coincidence, a poetic coincidence, but a coincidence nevertheless. After all, what you fail to take into account is the fact that Pete never once mentioned anything about something weird happening to him. And you know Peter, he's not exactly repressed." Larry Lawyer rests his case.

"I did take that into account. What *you* didn't take into account is the possibility that Peter did not experience a distinction between the real and the so-called unreal, the so-called normal and the paranormal. If there really is such a phenomenon as ESP, it seems to me that a person like Pete would be the most available to it and would probably not experience it as anything special."

"That's not a rational argument," Larry says not unkindly, "that's a belief. ESP is a mystery; unscientific, unexplained."

"So is gravity," I answer. "So what if we know that a falling object accelerates at a speed of thirty-two feet per second per second. What do we really know? We've just measured the mystery, that's all."

"Well," Larry concedes, "you're right about one thing. What happened today makes hope seem particularly seductive. Sometimes I wish I could believe in God. It would make all this somehow easier. Then maybe I'd see Peter's disease as having some purpose, some place in some scheme. At least there might be a chance that we could make some peace with it." He pounds one fist into the palm of the other. "I hate being so helpless. Oh Christ, I wish I believed in God, but I don't. I don't think I ever did. I could never believe with the others, the ones who stood at Grandpa Bill's grave, where a goddamn rug of plastic grass hid the hole. *'Adonai no-tan. Adonai lo-kah. Y'he sheym. Adonai m'vorach.'*

"I wish I could be like those old men. There they stood and still stand, for all I know—blessed, benighted—Christ, I don't know—declaring the impossible words of the faithful. 'The Lord giveth. The Lord taketh away. Blessed be the name of the Lord.' All I know is that I choked on those words then, and I choke on them now."

Tears are streaming down Larry's cheeks. He makes no move to brush them away. I do not dare touch his face or hand him a tissue.

"Oh, Larry! We must do something. This is an emergency! Peter is dying."

"There is nothing to do, except cultivate our garden. Take good care of each other, of Adam, of Peter. Do our best. This snake-oil faith we're fiddling with is dangerous. Not believing in God just makes you susceptible to crueler hoaxes. I know what's going on with you, Mary-Lou. Your brain is working overtime, rationalizing that if there's ESP, there must be such a thing as faith healing, and that Peter could be saved. You're already on your way to visit the fireman in England. And Esalen too. Am I right?"

"Yes," I mutter into my lap.

"I was too," he confesses. For a moment, neither of us speaks.

"We could go out to Esalen," I say at last. "The Junior Fellow program is about four months long. It'll be an adventure. Then we'd probably have to kill a few months before going to England. I think LeShan said it takes about a year to get an appointment with Chapman-Lang. We could spend the time in San Francisco. It's supposed to be a beautiful city. I've never been out West. We deserve it. Come on, Larry. Let's do it." I feel jumpy and dangerous inside, the way Eve must have felt when she offered Adam a bite.

"And have you also figured out how we're going to finance this little Looney Tunes toot of yours?"

"Couldn't we take a second mortgage on the house?"

"I suppose we could."

"And rent it for a year?"

"I guess so."

"And wouldn't your law firm pay you something while you're gone? I mean, they would be serving *your* clients. Isn't there something in the partnership agreement that allows for that?"

"I work for a law firm, not a university. Law firms don't give sabbaticals."

"They'd probably give you something each month, though, wouldn't they? That would only be fair."

"I suppose they would. They'd be fair."

"So between the money from the house and the law firm, we could make it, couldn't we?"

"You know what you, under any other circumstances, would call someone who thinks the way you are thinking, and hopes the way you are hoping?" Larry doesn't wait for me to answer. "You would call her 'pitiful.' "

"I would be right. I am pitiful. I even confess to being desperate. I know, or at least I nearly know, that Peter is doomed. But a piece of me resists. Part of me believes that something extraordinary happened today. I believe it because I believe in Pete, not because I trust my own fucked-up, cynical self. I believe in Pete's clarity, his light. I want to track this down. I want to see that healer in England. I want to try to do something for us by going to Esalen. I'm willing to take a chance on being proved a fool. I'm not willing to sit around here and watch us die."

Suddenly there is nothing I will not say. "What about us? What about you? What about the fact that we don't make love, really, anymore? What about what is happening to us? We need help as much as Peter."

"I'm suspicious of all that touchy-feely stuff, all those emotional explosions. It's not my way," Larry explains.

"Maybe you're just afraid of it. I know I am. Maybe our situation calls for some kicking and screaming. Let's have our privacy invaded for a change. Maybe we can exorcise the pain. I'm dying for a little mayhem."

"Or maybe we're just unwilling to grow up and face this."

"I'm not willing to grow up if growing up means giving up. I'm not willing to live without hope."

"Even if hope turns out to be as cruel as a peacock's eye?"

"It can't be any more cruel than this. Doing nothing is impossible. What have we got to lose? I don't even feel as if I'm making a choice."

"I know," Larry answers with resignation. And suddenly I understand that right now, together, we are loosing something powerful, reckless, alien and portentous into our lives. "That's what frightens me."

I can hear him practicing arpeggios inside. What have I come for? I think to myself. Daddy is never going to understand.

"Please do not ring the bell" reads a handwritten piece of note paper taped on the fluted, Doric door frame above the bell, at eye level. *"The noise disturbs the dog."*

I knock instead, death-rapping Beethoven's Fifth, our private code: a triplet of lights followed by one heavy. The music stops and I hear Impie begin to bark.

"Down, Impie, down, girl!" I hear my father scolding from indoors. "Don't worry," he says, opening the door with one hand, keeping the other on Impie's collar. "She won't hurt you. She just loves to announce the company."

I slip from the foyer into the living room like a thief while Impie bares her teeth at me in joyous welcome and strains to pull loose.

"If attacked by a wolf," reads *The Book of Emergencies,* the same book that suggests jumping up and down if caught in a plummeting elevator, "do not attempt to run. A wolf can outrun a human. Instead, lie down on the ground, roll onto your back, and bare your throat. Among the wolf species, this is the position of surrender. A wolf will rarely attack under those circumstances." For a panicky instant, I consider going belly up on the Kirman.

"If we sit down, I think she'll stop barking," says Daddy. "Now, what can I do for you?" he asks, looking up at me, smiling more with *pro forma* geniality than with affection. He seems to know I mean trouble. Impie lies folded at his feet, her head erect as if she were guarding a blind man on a bus.

I've decided not to tell him the whole truth. It would be crazy to tell him about Chapman-Lang. The only spirit Daddy has ever acknowledged is Hamlet's father's ghost.

I start boldly. "Larry and I have decided to take this next year off, rent the house and go to the Esalen Institute in Big Sur." I watch him closely. The next move is his. Daddy's hand travels toward his Phi Beta Kappa key. He begins to rub it between thumb and forefinger.

We are going to play a quick game of "Puritan Justice." I will be the plaintiff and the attorney for the plaintiff; he, in an even more dazzling display of virtuosity, will simultaneously play the roles of judge, prosecuting attorney, jury and, of course, hangman.

Released, the golden key falls back against a dark-gray herringbone vest. "And just what," Daddy asks, "do you hope to accomplish by so doing?" Sometimes I can sense, even before he is aware of it himself, the contempt in his voice. Loving him requires a slavish attention to nuance and detail. I can tell that he is holding the rat, the conversational rat, by the tail and at arm's length. Doomed; I can tell I am doomed. I should have known. I suppose I did.

"*Daddy? Daddy?*" *I know I am interrupting.*

"*What is it, Mary-Lou?*" *he winces, annoyed, turning away from the music stand, bow in hand, his head tucked down to hold the Stradivarius under his chin.*

"*Daddy,*" *I begin again, trying to summon some courage, even though I can tell already that I am lost, since whenever I interrupt him I am lost. But I plunge ahead to meet my fate.* "*Daddy, may I have a new dress for dancing school? I need one.*"

"*How many dresses do you have already?*" *he asks, patting the red welt on the side of his neck, where the violin rests, with his handkerchief.*

"*Two, I have two,*" *I say, already anticipating the course of the cross-examination,* "*but dancing school meets once each week for twenty weeks, and that means I have to wear the same dress ten times.*" *I plead my case, even though I know already, by the look on his face, that I have lost.*

"*Then,*" *he says triumphantly, tucking his handkerchief back into his pocket and lifting the Stradivarius to his waiting chin,* "*what you really mean is that you* want *a new dress.*" *He says* "*want*" *as if it were a dirty word.* "*Since you already* have *two dresses, you can't possibly* need *another dress, unless of course, both dresses are at the cleaners at the same time. Can you imagine any occasion when both dresses would be at the cleaners at the same time?*"

"*No,*" *I answer, just before the lump in my throat makes speech impossible. I hang my head in humiliation and defeat. I cannot tell him that what I really need is to feel pretty, to feel safe from all the boys at dancing school who will not ask me to dance because I am too tall, too smart, too snotty and too desperate. Irrelevant!*

"*Well, then . . .*" *he says, turning back to his music, placing the bow on the bridge. Sheriff! Take her away!*

I know all the evidence is against me, and still I persist, rushing toward his disapproval. "I'm not sure it's really a matter of what we 'hope to accomplish,' " I argue, trying to turn his own words against him by endowing their elocution with just a hint of rat's tail. "It's really that Larry and I are interested in Gestalt psychology, and we'd like to pursue that interest." In spite of my bravado I can hear my own voice, and I can tell that I am not convincing either of us, and that we both know it.

"So," he says, "because you are interested in Gestalt psychology, whatever that may be, you are going to uproot yourselves and your children, leave a lovely home, and Larry a perfectly good job with excellent opportunities, and go off into the wild blue yonder to live with hippies? That doesn't sound very responsible to me." Responsibility. The ultimate ethic. "It all sounds very self-indulgent to me." Self-indulgence. The cardinal sin. "But, of course, you don't need my permission," he finishes with a final twist, the psychological coup de grâce.

But I do need his approval. I do need his blessing. And he knows it. I will never stop knocking at his door, waiting, asking. Love me, Daddy. Take me in your arms. Dance me on your shoes.

"Look, Daddy," I say, knocking again, trying again. "It's not just because we're interested in Gestalt psychology. I don't know if you can understand this, but I feel very uninterested and bored with my life. I know that by all conventional standards we ought to feel contented, but we don't. Larry is bored with his practice, and I'm sick of being a housewife." I make very sure that I do not describe my condition as "unhappy." Daddy does not recognize happiness, or even the pursuit thereof, as one of the inalienable rights which we hold self-evident.

"We want to try something new. We want to find something better for ourselves. Maybe this is it. Maybe it isn't. If you're right, we'll find that out. All I know is that I have no more enthusiasm for the way we are living now." I stop, reeking of defeat, knowing that, as always, he has spotted the loophole in my argument, has slipped through it and is waiting for me on the other side.

"You're really talking about running away, and running away is irresponsible and indulgent, and if that were not enough, an affront to reason. You cannot honestly believe, Mary-Lou, that by running away to Esalen, or anywhere else for that matter, you can change anything!" He finishes with a rhetorical crescendo of disdain.

He is right! Goddamn it, he is right!

"You know, Mary-Lou," says Daddy with the understanding smile he saves for the vanquished, "I wouldn't be a bit surprised if you are confusing your frustration at not being able to do anything about Peter's condition with what you call 'boredom.' " A brilliant and noble judge! A jewel on the bench.

The tears that form in my eyes amount to a confession and a plea. You are right. I cannot honestly believe that I can change anything by running away, that I can save my own life, or Peter's; I'm too much like you. But, oh God, I must try!

Oh, Daddy, please find a way to stop me if I am wrong, to spare me, ahead of time, if I am going to be hurt. Do you understand? I can't stop myself. I'm not like you that way. You just need to be right. I want to be happy.

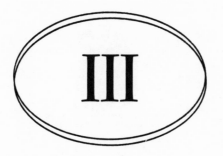

III

I do my thing and you do your thing. I am not in this world to
live up to your expectations. And you are not in this world to
live up to mine. You are you and I am I, and if by chance we
find each other, it's beautiful. If not, it can't be helped.

Frederick S. Perls

Adam is reading aloud from the poster tacked to the wall in
the tiny, rough-hewn Esalen office where we are waiting our
turn to register.

"I really like that quote," Larry says. "It's refreshing,
don't you think?" After all his previous skepticism, Larry has
arrived gung ho. I seem to have spent all my enthusiasm getting here.

"I don't know," I answer slowly, releasing my words, one
by one, like hostages. "Something about it bothers me."

"What?"

"I'm not sure. Something. Maybe it's that it sounds too callous."

"It sounds pretty nice to me." Larry shifts Peter in his arms, gives him a quick kiss on the side of the neck and whispers conspiratorially in his ear, "Your mommy's a funny lady, Pete. Even the possibility of happiness makes her nervous. It's the Russian in her." I hate it when he tells the kids on me.

"No, it's not," I respond. "It's the *Jew* in me. The Russian only aids and abets. Jews have a special mission."

"And what's that?"

"Never to be comfortable in the world."

"And if Mommy ever *did* feel at home, God forbid," Larry adds into Peter's ear, "she would think it somehow shameful."

Maybe he's right. Maybe it's not some ethical imperative, this discomfort of mine, but some perverse will to set myself apart, to think too much, to hover over my life like a balloon over the Macy's Thanksgiving Day parade, casting a grotesque shadow that only I can see.

I tuck myself away in one corner of the office and look out the window at this new world. In the distance the plush green mountains stack against each other and the sky. Like heavy folds of Renaissance skirts, they slide toward the sea, their hems dipping, then disappearing, in the mist rising off the Pacific. The fierce sun, flat and fluid as a dish of blood, begins to eclipse behind the horizon, making the sky glow and dyeing the ocean pink.

Esalen rests in a shallow valley on one of these promontories, as if held over the ocean in the palm of a giant hand.

Life is in bloom. Flowers sip through stems so exquisitely succulent they would split open and spill at the touch of a fingernail. Bunches of daisies sprout at optimistic angles from mossy crannies in stone garden walls. Spongy, voluptuous lawns, watered to a pampered green by mists, roll gently downhill from the mountains into this verdant declivity, and then slightly uphill, coming to a ragged surprise ending at the edge of the cliff.

On the side of the hill, young men and women wearing red and blue bandannas tied around their heads lean into shovels in a garden so yeasty with organic richness that the dark soil rises and crumbles like cake around each cut of the spade.

Near a stand of tattered, romantic eucalyptus trees, a group of people shyly picks partners. They hold each other's hands like children going to recess. They are taking turns at being blind. The sighted partners tug gentle encouragement. Come. Trust me. The blind lean backward in their soft tracks, or grope with their one free hand, as sleepwalkers are supposed to do. They pat the sides of trees.

They lead and are led, trust and are trusted, depend and are dependable, take control and give it up. Every once in a while somebody whose turn it is to be blind giggles nervously, perhaps dismissing as crazy the thought that comes unwelcome to his mind—that this trusted stranger to whom he clings might just push him off the cliff.

Near the edge of the cliff a bare-chested man with hair and beard as long as a prophet's stands stock-still on one foot in a jewel of light and raises the other foot ceremoniously in front of him, keeping it bent. With his arms he reaches slowly at the sky, as if he would wring its neck.

"What's the man doing, Mommy?" It's Adam.

"I don't know, sweetie. It looks like some kind of a dance."

"It's *tai chi.*" The young woman who has been bent forward over registration forms at the counter turns to answer. Her long brown hair, as eternal as Eve's, falls past her slim shoulders. She wears a purple leotard. Just below her molded waist, from the barely detectable place where the swell of her belly begins, a skirt of Indian fabric hangs straight to the floor.

She is not wearing a bra. Beneath the leotard, the nipples of her young, full breasts are well-defined, yet intriguingly distorted, like the nylon-stockinged faces of holdup men. They sway slightly in the wake of her sudden turn. Larry's eyes follow them as if they were the eyes of Christ in a storefront window. I am unattractive out West.

"It's not really a dance. It's more like a meditative exercise. Hi," she adds, "my name's Felicity Plum. Are you waiting to register for the Junior Fellow program?"

"Yes." Larry finds his voice and then loses it.

I pitch in. "He's Larry. And this is Adam and this is Peter, and I'm Mary-Lou. Hi." My hand sticks out long enough in the air before she takes it to convince me that shaking is not "in" out here. I am middle-aged out West.

"What workshops are you signing up for?" Felicity asks.

"Whatever the Junior Fellow program is, that's what we'll be taking," I answer.

"You get to choose," says Felicity, "from the regular catalog."

"But I thought there was going to be a special—"

"Sounds great!" says Larry. "What do you recommend?"

" 'The Experience of Esalen' is supposed to be terrific."

"Is Betty Fuller leading it?" I ask.

"Oh, you guys know Betty Fuller too? No, unfortunately, she's not. Isn't she outrageous? God, I love that woman! She's like a mother to me. Really. The first time I worked with Betty—it was at an Esalen workshop in San Francisco—I didn't have any idea of what to expect. What a woman!

"First, she kicks open the door like a cowboy, and there she is in her flowered mumu, all two-hundred and eighty pounds of her, her hands held out in front of her like drawn six-shooters . . ." Felicity puffs up her slight self, looks tough, kicks open an imaginary saloon door, hitches up her skirt with her elbows and twirls her imaginary guns at us. "And then she hollers, 'Okay, motherstickers, this is a fuck-up!' "

I smile and wait and watch my shadow lengthen and grow dark while Larry and Felicity and Adam and Peter laugh together.

"Is Betty here now?" I ask. "I can't wait to see her."

"She's here, but you probably won't see her until group."

"Tonight's group?"

"I don't think so. She's finishing up a week-long acupuncture workshop and the party's tonight. She'll be leading the group tomorrow night, and then for the rest of the week. After that she'll be splitting her time between San Francisco and Big Sur."

"I thought she was going to be here all the time!"

"Calm down, Mary-Lou." Larry sounds annoyed. I am spoiling his fun. "Betty's going to be here, just not all of the time. She never *said* she was going to be here all of the time, did she?"

"No, I guess not, I just assumed—"

"Are you people here to register?" A bearded young man looks up from his work behind the counter. His brown beard is soft and scraggly like a Hasid's, as if he's never shaved, but his cheek is as tan and glowing as a surfer's. He wears denim overalls. The tag on the bib reads: "Oshkosh B'gosh."

"We're the Weismans," says Larry, getting down to business.

"You're the people with the kids?" He looks up from the forms.

"Right," says Larry.

"Far out!"

"All the way from Connecticut!" I quip. Nobody laughs. I am not funny out West.

"This is the first time that Esalen is allowing non-staff people with kids, so keep them mellow, all right?"

"They're good kids—aren't you, guys?" I move in toward the children, touching each instinctively, as if to soothe the betrayal of my words.

"We thought we'd do 'The Experience of Esalen' workshop." Larry plunges his hands into his pockets like a cowboy.

"Wait a minute, Larry! Don't you think it's probably a lot like what we did at the Bucks County Seminar House?"

"If Betty's not leading the group, it's bound to be another experience—the Gestalt will be altogether different." Larry's speech pattern is changing before my ears.

"Okay." My shadow lengthens. "If you think so."

"That way," says the young man at the desk, "you can take the couples group in the evening."

A dread sensation of free fall in my gut lets me know that I do not want to take the couples group. Nevertheless, I nod my head in happy unison when Larry says, "Sure. Why not?" Larry is existential. Larry is human potential.

"Would you like to be in the same couples group, or would you prefer splitting up, doing the workshop at different times and with different people?"

If we take the group together, I will never tell, and Larry will never say, "I can't have an orgasm." I look to Larry and join the chorus. "Same group. Whatever."

"You'll be staying at South Coast with the rest of the Junior Fellows. We've assigned you two rooms, 105 and 107. South Coast is the motel facility that you passed about a mile up Route One on your left on your way down here."

I panic at the idea of Peter released in so much undomesticated space, weary on the road, overwhelmed by the mountains, threatened by the cliffs. "Are the rooms connected?"

"You mean from the inside?"

"Yes."

"No, they're not."

"No problem! No problem!" Larry hastens to reassure. "Adam can just holler or bang on the wall if he needs us. No problem." Larry is laid-back. Larry is California.

"Don't worry about the kids," Felicity volunteers. "This place is a paradise for kids. They'll be very happy and safe here. There's plenty of space to play. They've got the pool, the sauna, the gardens, the baths, the mountains—what could be better?"

Maybe she didn't notice. "I worry about Peter." I touch the top of Peter's head gently. "Pete's got a muscle problem," I say as cheerfully as possible, to discourage her from getting all upset, just in case she's one of those who, when I tell them, act as if they did it, as if it were their fault. "He falls a lot, and *some*times when he falls"—I tell it slightly singsong, like a favorite story that Peter has requested at many bedtimes—"*some*times he can't get up!" The "he can't get up" part is said like a surprise ending, the way you'd say "happily ever after."

"Well, you won't have to worry here." Felicity smiles at Peter. "You aren't back East anymore where people are such uptight assholes that they don't care about anyone else but themselves." Peter smiles back at her.

"Esalen is a *real* community. It's not like any other place you know. It's a caring, cooperative community. We all help in the gardens and in the kitchen. We're available to one another. If Peter should fall and you're not there, someone will pick him up."

"Just like that?" I ask. I feel my dry, withered spirit dare to dampen and dilate.

"Just like that." Felicity touches my arm gently with her hand.

"That would be nice," I say, feeling tears form in my eyes.

"What did you do today in school?" I call to the kids as they cross the lawn to meet me. Even after three months I find myself keeping to my East Coast maternal patterns, even though out here there is no school bus, no group of mothers waiting at the end of the street in curlers, no lunch boxes. Pete carries a crayoned drawing by one corner, and Adam is holding what looks like a composition rolled into a cylinder. There is no kitchen table to sit at. There are no milk and cookies, either.

"C'mere, guys. Let me see what you've got there."

Adam swaggers over, doing his Big Sur cowboy walk, in cut-off jeans, fringed vest and the ever present Buck knife in its leather scabbard, tied to his thigh with a piece of rawhide. "I need it," he had argued when Larry and I questioned the propriety of an eight-year-old with a real knife, a sharp knife, "for cutting through the Big Sur wilderness. There might," he had advised us, his eyes glistening with solemnity, "be bears."

Peter lurches toward me, sway-backed, pigeon-toed. Scraped knees mean he has been falling. The disease is surfacing. It is time for a wheelchair.

"I wonder what this could be. . . ." I put on my present-opening voice, relieving Peter of the drawing. There is no refrigerator door to hang the picture on, either. "Now, let's see. What is it?" I point. "What are all these red rickracks over here?"

"It's a song called Beethoven's Ninth," says Pete.

"Pete's class drew to music today," Adam explains.

"It's a terrific picture," I say to Pete.

"It's a song picture. The black scribbles are when the music got dark."

"The black scribbles are very nice too," I add.

"Is that a composition you've got, Adam?" I ask. "What's it about? May I see it?"

"It's a fucking composition," Peter says. "Adam's class wrote fucking compositions," he adds, as if he has somehow clarified the matter for both of us.

Confused, curious, I unroll the paper. It is entitled "The Fucking Composition." I begin to read.

"This fucking girl and this fucking boy were walking down to the fucking baths together, when the fucking boy said to the fucking girl, let's fuck. And so they did. They fucked, and they fucked again, and they fucked again. They fucked three times."

"What the—what the heck is this supposed to be?" I am surprised, caught flat-footed, somewhere on the way between laughter and anger, my destination still undetermined.

"My teacher assigned it," Adam explains. "She said we were all saying the f-word too much, so she made us write this composition."

"As a punishment?" I ask, seeking familiar, reassuring territory. I am not quite sure of how to be, who to be, who is me—the eccentric East Coast matron, or the West Coast Geritol hippie.

"Kind of a punishment, but not exactly," Adam answers. "She said we should get it out of our systems. She said that it was Gestalt to exaggerate something bad, to get it out of your system. She said we each had to use it in a story ten times. I won. I used it eleven times; once for extra credit."

"Far out!" I laugh, thinking to myself, You can take the kid out of the East, but you can't take the East out of the kid. Or his mother, for that matter. "I'll see you guys later. I've got a group in the baths."

I tousle Adam's hair and kneel to hug Peter. "Snurgle flop, puny blaster, grungle, grungle, grungle," I mutter behind his ear before releasing him, pausing a moment with my hands perched lightly on the sway of his back, to make sure he has regained his balance.

"Are you planted?" I ask.

"Like a petunia," he answers.

"Okay, petunia puss."

"Mom?"

"What, Petie?"

"How come every time you go away, a sad place grows in my tummy?"

"Probably because we love each other," I answer, feeling a sad place grow in mine.

"Or maybe," says Peter, "it's because I don't want you to go away."

"What the fuck am I doing here?" I mutter to myself as I climb the path to the baths.

We are sitting shoulder to shoulder like missionaries in a cauldron, five to a tub, in sulfuric water so hellishly hot as to be almost unbearable. Someone has brought a transistor radio to the baths. The sounds of classical music are punctuated by occasional staccato yelps of pain and of relief as some bathers stand up to escape the heat, while others lower themselves into the hot water to escape the chill of the November air. Fall has come to paradise.

My lungs labor to accept the dull stench of sulfur, mixed with the insinuating sweet of burning incense and rising steam. Although totally nude, we are disembodied heads, floating like surreal Magrittes above the gray, glassy water. Our bodies and limbs, submerged and distorted beneath the water's surface, seem broken, irrelevant, askew. Touchingly helpless, yet fetal and repellent, like chicken parts in a roiling pot, our dead-white, incandescent joints founder with buoyancy in the gray cement tubs.

"Rub-a-dub-dub, one man and two women in a tub," Felicity giggles. I am looking through the water at the tops of her feet. Tiny chains of bubbles cling to the fine blonde hairs which protrude and wave like exotic ferns on the ocean's floor.

"You know what?" I ask Larry.

"I'll tell you what," Larry fires back. "I wish that just once you would say something straight out, without having to say 'You know what' before you deliver yourself of the message. It's as if you're about to perform and you want to get the audience's attention. Why must you always act as if you are for sale?"

"Is that what you've learned about me so far at Esalen?" I challenge, unable fully to deflect either the truth of his remark or the pain that it has caused me.

"That, and one additional fact—that you don't have any scruples about taking your clothes off in public. You got undressed over there"—he cocks his head, indicating the hooks on the wall near the massage tables—"like Gypsy Rose Lee."

"Actually," I defend myself, "what I was about to say after I so illegitimately captured your attention is that I am surprised that Esalen is such an unsexy place. You'd think with all this nudity, all these breasts, the acres of flourishing pubic hair, you'd think you'd see at least a few erect penises."

"That's probably," Larry snaps, "because most of the women have the men's balls in their pockets."

"May I join you?" asks a stranger with closely trimmed sideburns and pale-blue boxer shorts. He inquires with the civilized reticence of a solitary moviegoer who arrives just after the lights have gone out and wonders if the empty seat next to you, where you have parked your coat, is taken.

"My name is Larry," says Larry, extending a steaming, dripping hand.

"My name is Roger. I just got here this afternoon with the IBM junior executive training program."

"Nice to meet you, Roger," says Larry, grinning broadly. "Why don't you take your shorts off and stay a while?"

"That's okay," says Roger, smiling and embarrassed, "I feel strange taking my pants off."

"A lot of people are like that at first. In a couple of days you'll feel strange with your pants on. Now, take my wife, for instance ..." Larry gestures in my direction. "She's only been here three months and she just loves to take her pants off."

"Larry, please stop! I hate this!" I cry.

Larry looks about desperately for a moment and buries his head in his hands. "I'm sorry. Forgive me."

"It's all right," I lie.

"Really?" Larry implores.

"Really."

"I don't believe either of you," Felicity challenges amiably. "Since we all do what we want to do, I invite you to own up to wanting to hurt Mary-Lou." Larry reaches for his cigarettes on the ledge of the tub. "And now, Larry, you're going to piss away your feelings in smoke. And as for you," she adds, turning with great determination toward me, "I invite you to consider the possibility that you don't forgive Larry, especially not 'really.' If he had said that about me, I wouldn't feel forgiving. You know, Mary-Lou, you poison yourself with bad feelings when you don't let them out."

"I don't want to let them out," I answer stubbornly. I can feel them gnawing at my chest.

"Okay, just so long as you take responsibility for not being willing to share your feelings with us. You realize, of course, that by refusing to work on these feelings, you are really holding the rest of us hostage emotionally. You have all the power."

She is absolutely right. I sit sullen, silent, with my jaw set, my arms wrapped tightly around my knees, relishing resentment and contempt as they eat their way into my chest.

"I feel sad that Mary-Lou is unwilling to trust us with her true feelings. How do you feel about this?" Felicity calls on Larry.

"I take responsibility for hurting Mary-Lou," he mumbles, as if there were a gun to his head.

"Why don't you tell her—she's sitting right next to you," Felicity prompts with an encouraging smile.

Reluctantly Larry turns toward me. He looks very tired and very uncomfortable.

"Remember to make eye contact," Felicity coaches.

"I can take responsibility for hurting you, Mary-Lou. I can't say that I didn't mean to. I obviously did mean to, or I wouldn't have done it. Right now, I'm not in touch with the part of me that wants to hurt you. I'm only aware of the part that's sorry."

"Beautiful, Larry. That was really beautiful. Now, what about you? Do you have anything you want to share with Mary-Lou?" Felicity nods at Roger.

"Well," says Roger, "I just met her . . . I just got here this afternoon, but"—he pauses for a moment before turning toward me, "you seem like a very nice person, Mary-Lou. I hope you feel better soon."

"Thank you, Roger" is all I can say before my throat tightens, but I wonder how come the only person I believe is a square from IBM who sounds like a Hallmark greeting card.

* * *

Key-locked, key-locked, key-locked, key-locked is the sound my spoon makes against the inside of the white, ceramic coffee mug. I stir briskly, trying to melt off the reluctant amber blob of honey. Sugar is not served in the dining hall at Esalen. "Fucking honey," I mumble at my spoon.

"Hold it, everybody! Hold it!" Dan, who is sitting next to me, sets down his knife and fork. "I think Mary-Lou has another little resentment she'd like to share with the group. Something else here does not altogether meet with her approval. Mary-Lou, would you care to express . . ."

I am alert to a familiar hazard. I am in enemy territory. They lie in wait everywhere—in vats of hot water, behind pillows, in the dining hall, watching for a breach in my rational, front-line defenses. At the first indication of weakness, they will sound the battle cry, *Charge!*, and fall upon me. They want to capture my feelings. They want to drink my blood.

After four months of breakdowns and breakthroughs, we are addicted to a steady diet of fresh feelings. Wasted, diddled nearly insensate by our own and one another's tales of child abuse, premature ejaculation, compulsive eating and frigidity, which we re-enact as if they were charades, we primal yentas keep shuffling the cards, upping the ante, going for broke.

Here it is always Shrove Tuesday. We wear our emotional insides out, like huge papier-mâché caricatures at Mardi Gras, and celebrate them in the streets like the Seven Deadly Sins.

"Fuck off, Dan." Felicity intervenes on my behalf. "We're supposed to be planning a farewell party. It's just not going to happen unless we all take responsibility for making it happen. Claude, you're taking care of the main course, right?"

"I was thinking maybe chicken . . ." Claude lounges back in his chair. Midway through yesterday's evening group, while we were doing some bioenergetic breathing, Claude claims to have re-experienced his own birth. Nobody believed him.

"It was a *good* rebirth," Dan had joked, walking over to shake hands with the bawling, red-faced Claude, "but not a *great* rebirth. I give it three stars."

"Four stars," Larry had offered, "if you eat the placenta."

"I can make pâté out of the livers," Molly offers, delicately touching the damp tip of her tongue to the tiny pile of sunflower seeds which rests in her palm. In the psychodrama workshop, Molly tied up her incestuous father and then cut him up into small but still eloquently describable pieces.

"Author! Author!" Dan had called, applauding, from his cross-legged perch on top of a pillow.

"I'll make some French bread," Larry volunteers as he swings his legs over the arm of his chair and lights up a cigarette. "And it won't be whole wheat, either."

"I need my roughage," says Dan.

"How about apple juice for the drink?" Felicity suggests.

"Far fuckin' out!" Bernice approves. "And we'll spike it with LSD."

"Just a little," says Molly with a smile.

"Now you're talking," says Dan.

"You guys are kidding, aren't you? You're not going to put LSD in the apple juice?" I'm almost positive they're kidding. Even though Bernice made a play for an Arab proctologist in the "Divorce as a Creative Experience" workshop and went swimming at South Coast in her biofeedback equipment, she is still a sixty-year-old woman from Yonkers. That's got to count for something.

"I'm not kidding," she insists. "We'll tell everybody it's spiked, of course. That way, it'll be their choice. Don't worry, Mary-Lou, we're not going to *force* you to drink it."

"What about the kids?" I hear my voice go shrill.

"Oh, Jeezus!" Bernice rolls her eyes at Dan. "She thinks I've forgotten about the kids. How *could* we forget the little darlings," she implores everyone at the table. "The mother superior here wouldn't let us. Don't worry"—she reaches across the table to patronize me on the arm—"we won't let the good kids have any of the bad juice, okay?"

"No, it's not okay." Now I am really screaming. "What if one of the kids wanders by and picks up a cup someone has left around with a little bit still at the bottom, and the kid drinks it—"

"For Chrissakes," Bernice laughs. "I was only kidding. Can't you take a joke? Wow! Are you ever on a heavy mother trip."

Something has gone wrong; terribly, terribly wrong. It was not supposed to turn out like this. I have never known so many people so well and liked them so little. I have never been known so well by so many people and been so disliked.

"We'd better clear the table . . ." Felicity fills the silence while I swallow my anger. "There's a group tonight at eight."

"Eight! Oh, shit, is it almost eight?" I exclaim. "I've got to find the kids and tuck them in."

"Tuck the kids in?" Bernice asks in the rhetorical rat-by-the-tail tone. "You've got to lay off those kids. You're too uptight. Peter will be just fine," she says with much exasperation. "When children get sleepy, they just lie down and go to sleep. Kids are wonderful that way. They just naturally know how to take care of themselves. Kids are very mellow, in-touch people. If I could control you, I would have you give yourself permission to relax and let the kids be."

"She's right, honey," says Larry, who loves to hang around the dining hall after dinner, reminiscing about his days in the rat race until it's time to climb the hill to our evening workshop. "Relax. Hang loose. So what if they fall asleep under a tree?"

"I can't relax, Larry. That's just the point." I can feel my throat constricting, my eyes filling.

"Not can't—won't," says Larry, lighting up another cigarette.

I don't know which one of them I can't stand more—Bernice or Larry, with their supercilious I'm-more-laid-back-than-thou attitude.

"Come on, Larry," I plead. "Help me find Adam and Pete

and put them to bed." I hate to hear myself begging. "Please!" I add, getting up and pushing my chair under the table.

"Come on yourself," he says, turning to rest his feet defiantly on my chair. "It's your problem. If you feel you must tuck the kids into bed, by all means, do your own thing; but don't try to hijack me on your guilt trip."

"Are you serious?" is all I can say before tears threaten.

"Yup," says Larry. He puckers up and releases a perfect smoke ring.

"Fuck you, Larry, oh, fuck you!" I yell, hitting him square in the jaw with my fist. I scarcely acknowledge the pain that is shooting through my arm as I watch Larry, stupefied, wipe the blood from his lip with the back of his hand.

"Far out," I hear Bernice gasp as I turn and rush through the dining hall toward the door. "Far fuckin' out!"

My body sweating, my brain swarming with anger and pain, I run across the carefully tended law, feeling the grass springy beneath my feet. I slow down at the garden, now dense with vegetables that grow as fast as pods in science fiction. "Adam! Peter!" I call into the dark, leafy fecundity. No answer.

I plunge up the hill toward the cabins. I open door after door, pausing only to call inside, "Adam! Peter!" One by one, interrupted faces look up from books, from conversations, from behind smoke and reorganize themselves to say "No."

Maybe they're talking to the gate guard. I run through the parking lot toward the gate guard's hut. I should have thought of that first. They love to talk to the gate guards.

"Have you seen Adam and Peter?" It is Larry's voice asking. He is already at the guard shack.

"They haven't been around here."

There are only two places left—the cliffs and the baths. "You check the cliffs," I call to Larry over my shoulder. "I'll check the baths." I double back across the lawn, past the stone walls and the daisies, past the flowering bushes serenely topped by scores of migrating monarch butterflies. Soon it will be winter in paradise.

I am stalking tragedy now. Almost confident of it. I dig my heels into the dusty path that winds down to the baths. Adam would have to have held Peter's hand to slow him down. The gray cement tubs skulk out of the cliffside like concrete bunkers on the Normandy shore.

No one is there. The steam rises, mixes with the cold mist and the punk of burning incense and nudges up against the gray cinder-block walls. A reptilian-green vinyl hose lies coiled, drooling a weak stream of cold water onto the concrete floor. A foil-bright red-white-and-blue can of Ajax shines in the moonlight.

Desperate, I head for the cliffs. I press my toes into the dirt and lean in, running against the hill. As I round the crest and head out toward the cliffs I see Larry's body, dark as a shadow but substantial, against the sky. He sees me, too, and motions to me: Go slow—be quiet—hush! As I move slowly forward, I hear the sound of a child's voice.

"Shit! Fuck! Milk! Cookies! Shit! Fuck! Milk! Cookies!" It is Peter. Thank God, it is Peter. Through the darkness I see him on the ground near the cliff's edge, alternately yelling and pounding, punching his little fists enthusiastically, if ineffectually, into a huge pillow. Adam, his hands on his hips, presides close by. "Shit! Fuck! Milk! Cookies! I don't think it's working, Adam. I don't feel any different except that my throat hurts."

"Don't worry about it," says Adam. "It never works for me, either. Try one more time, and then we'll quit for tonight. Mom's probably looking for us."

"Shit! Fuck! Milk! Cookies!" Peter cries once more into the cold, starry night before flinging himself, sobbing, onto the pillow. "It doesn't work, Adam. I still hate it here."

"Adam?" Larry's voice is soft. "It's Daddy. Peter is a little too close to the edge. Please help him move away. Do it nice and easy; that's right . . . no big deal . . ." He talks them toward safety. "Good boy."

"Don't ever go so close to the edge again!" I scold, kneeling to hug them around the silky backs of their knees, anger leaking out around the edges of relief.

"C'mon, guys." Larry lifts Peter up in his arms.

"Where are we going?" Pete sniffs.

"Well," says Larry, "tonight we're all going intobedyougo early."

"And then what," says Adam.

"And then, tomorrow, we're all getting the hell out of here."

Sit down, for Chrissakes! For Chrissakes, Pete, stop walking and get into that wheelchair. Get into that wheelchair. Get used to that wheelchair. God! Make him get into the wheelchair, for Chrissakes.

Peter is pushing his wheelchair up Telegraph Hill as if it were a walker, and I am clenching my teeth and screaming into my brain.

"You've been pushing that wheelchair all over San Francisco. Why don't you give yourself a break, Pete," says Larry. "Climb in and I'll give you a free ride." I marvel at how instinctively and humanely right he is about Pete and hate myself for not being able to feel beyond my anger.

"Let *me* push, Daddy. Let *me* push Pete. After all, he's *my* brother," Adam urges, adding, "he's just *your* kid. Right, Pete?" Adam's adaptive love makes him seem old, one of us.

"I don't want to get in," Pete insists, his pudgy hands gripping the dove-gray rubberized handles on the red vinyl wheelchair, junior model. His body leans in toward the wheelchair at a perilous angle, straining tiptoe against the collective forces of gravity, the big chrome wheels and the discouraging incline of the hill. "I don't want to get in. I want to give Adam a ride."

"Okay," says Adam, flashing Larry a conspiratorial glance. "First *you* push *me,* and then I'll push *you.* Is that a deal?"

We pause alongside an old goatherd's bungalow set into the hill, flush against the road. Salmon-colored geraniums bloom in the window box. Its frame and haphazard shingles, once painted a hard Arles blue, now chalky and faded, seem to be struggling to find a level foothold amid the curve of the roadway, the concave grace of the Golden Gate Bridge, and the oblique roof lines of vertical Victorians set into the parabolic hills.

Larry braces his hip against the back of the wheelchair while Adam sits down. Pete intensifies his grip on the handles, his face almost steamy with exertion. Even Larry is panting. "Christ," he says, "this headache is a doozie."

"Did you know that Telegraph Hill used to be a goat pasture?" I ask.

"I didn't know it, but I believe it," says Larry. "This is certainly a better goat hill than a people hill, don't you think so, boys? This sure is no city for old men," he recites in my direction, bastardizing Yeats.

Or cripples, either.

"I suppose we ought to take the apartment we saw on Vallejo Street, the one near Van Ness," I say.

I hate it. I don't want to live in it. It is not a San Francisco house. It isn't even a San Francisco apartment. Gold flecks twinkle in a plaster ceiling, painstakingly troweled to an overlapping fan pattern. Orange wall-to-wall with nubby bumps makes the place look like a motel. S&H Green Stamp colonial furniture and the Etruscan caryatids in the lobby, with grapes on their heads, make matters worse. We might as well be in Des Moines.

"*This* is a nice goat house," says Peter, reaching out one hand to touch the shaggy blue shingles. "I want to live in this tippy house."

"The apartment on Vallejo is a good location," Larry agrees. "It's on a flat street, no stairs from the sidewalk to the lobby, an elevator . . . and it's furnished. I don't think we can do any better. Why don't we stop looking and take it. The rent's not too bad and we can have it without a lease, on a month-to-month basis."

"And you didn't even mention the gold flecks in the ceiling. Do you think the landlord would let us put a flamingo on the lawn?" I can't believe how horrible I am being.

"I like the gold flecks," says Peter. "They're like stars."

"What do you have against flamingos?" Adam asks.

"I'm sorry, you guys. Your mother is a doo-doo," I confess, liberating a little love from my mean heart.

"Cheer up, Mary-Lou. Don't be such a brat. This is going to be a great adventure. Six months in the most beautiful city in America with nothing that we have to do, no work to go to, not a single obligation except to keep an appointment in eight months with the schizophrenic fireman in England—a fitting end to your California experience. Enjoy it."

I am convinced I should be happy. Sulking in my shoes, I am having none of it.

"Come on," Larry tries again. "Get some of those California vibes going. When in San Francisco . . . relax. Lighten up, mellow out, save the whales."

"Okay," I laugh, breaking my bonds, "as long as I don't have to have a nice day."

"Come on, Pete," says Larry, "the troops are rested. Let's push Adam to the top of the hill."

"It's not fair that we have to go to school," says Adam as soon as we are moving again. "It's against kids' rights. Besides, it's already January. It's too late to start school. It could be traumatic for us," he adds darkly from his perch on the wheelchair.

"Do you know what 'traumatic' means?" I delight in his high-speed mind and con-man delivery.

"It means what Daddy said about the playground at my new school yesterday when we went to visit—a cross between Hong Kong harbor and Muhammad Ali's training camp."

"What did you mean, Larry?"

"I meant that the mix in Adam's new school is one-third white, one-third Oriental and one-third black. San Francisco has just instituted busing. It may be a little rough for you at first, Adzie, but I think you're going to like it."

"Why are they called black when they're brown?" asks Peter.

"I don't really know, Fudgetickle. Some black people, especially in Africa, where they originally came from, are almost black. They want to be called black, so I guess that's a good enough reason, even if they aren't exactly black."

"We're not exactly white either," says Peter, scrutinizing his arm. "I'm more exactly pink, with brown freckles and white hairs and some other dots that I'm not sure what they are. Can I go to Adam's school?" says Pete, still pushing. "Why can't I go to Adam's school?"

This time I am ready. I rehearsed last night under the motel shower. I can feel the soothing water beating down on my head now as I repeat myself: "Because this school is designed especially for you and for kids like you who have muscle problems or other problems, like having to wear braces on their legs or needing crutches, and stuff like that. Your school doesn't have any stairs, and a bus will pick you up right in front of our apartment."

It is one of those times when I hear my own voice, see my own words, reeled out from me like laundry, hung with clothespins on the line. I sound to myself as earnestly optimistic as a Girl Scout troop leader in a nuclear holocaust with my act-as-if-nothing-is-happening voice, as if Sunshine School children were lucky children, the luckiest, fittest children in spite of "needing crutches, and stuff like that"; oh yes, the most elected-to-survive children, the most-likely-to-succeed children—Darwinism as yearbook lingo—and not the maimed or the mutant, selected out to follow some haywire, genetic command to eat themselves alive. But Peter will not be conned.

"I can climb stairs and I can even go up great big hills."

"But sometimes you fall and get hurt." I can tell that I am handling this all wrong, that I cannot handle this, that I cannot knowingly set out to break my own child's spirit, nor can I collude with him in clinging to the fantasy that he is normal until he, quite literally, drops in his tracks. Nor do I see another way.

"Listen, kiddo, listen, ol' Fudgetickle Entworth LaRue, this is an order. You are to go to the Sunshine School and like it, or else," Larry threatens, baring his teeth.

"Or else what?" Pete challenges saucily.

"Or else I'll bite your nose off!" Larry shoots right back, his eyes twinkling. With one more tortured, pressed macadam step, we round the crest of Telegraph Hill. Adam climbs out of the wheelchair.

"Now shut up and get in the wheelchair. It's your turn!" Larry commands like a low-comedy corporal, never losing the cadence. "Hop in, kid." And Pete hops right in.

A kid in a wheelchair. He looks almost normal. It is just now Wednesday, January 5, 1972, 11:30 A.M. And we are a family taking a walk.

"There's Coit Tower," says Adam. "It looks like a dickie." And the boys start laughing.

"For Chrissakes, you guys," I protest. "Whoever taught you to call a penis a dickie!" But they just keep giggling.

"Stop laughing, you loonies. This is your mother speaking. First of all, Coit Tower does *not* look like a penis. It looks like exactly what it's supposed to look like. It's a replica of a firehose nozzle. It was erected by some lady to commemorate the San Francisco firemen."

"Erected, you say?" says Larry, giving it to me in the ribs.

"Fire hoses look like dickies," says Adam.

"It's incredible, isn't it?" I question the air. "You hang Matisse mobiles in front of their faces the minute they come home from the hospital; you stimulate their brains—and deaden yours—with one-way conversations; you play Bach on the stereo and try to engender self-respect by insisting upon addressing the parts of the human anatomy by their proper names—breasts, penis, vagina—not Mrs. Breasts, not Mommy's boobs or headlights, and certainly not Mr. Penis, or Daddy's dickie—and what do you get? Kids who won't stop talking, love rock music and call their penises 'dickies.' That's what you get! I can't stand it another minute!" I begin to run pell-mell out of control down the other side of Telegraph Hill, laughing. I hear Petie's voice grow louder behind me. "Faster, Adam, faster! Push me faster! Let's catch Mommy!"

The wheelchair careens past us at the bottom of the hill.

Larry! They're going to crash! I want to yell, but my voice has turned to bone in my throat.

"Slow down!" Larry calls, just as Adam takes his leg off the strut, stretches it backwards, drags his foot like an anchor along the road while steering the wheelchair in a wide arc, bringing it to a stop with a scraping flourish alongside us.

Fear vibrates behind my ribs like a cold brass cymbal. "For Chrissakes, Adam, you could have killed him!"

"Go a little more slowly, Adzie-babe," says Larry. "We don't want either of you hurt."

"Can we do it again, Adam, can we?" Pete pleads.

The neural ringing in my chest subsides. I catch an unpleasant glimpse of myself, desperate, fearful, dangerously, ineluctably, bone-to-bone, muscle-to-muscle, connected blood-to-blood, to Peter.

"Take it easy, Mary-Lou. They weren't in any real danger. Besides, Pete loves it."

"I think I'm turning into a nervous wreck," I mutter. "I'm worried about myself."

"Don't worry. Lighten up," Larry answers, patting me on the hand. "Come on, youze guys. Let's proceed down this street in an orderly fashion. There seems to be a big crowd a few blocks down. Let's investigate."

"Don't worry, you say? What a good idea! I'm amazed that I didn't think of that myself. Do you have any more good advice?"

"As a matter of fact, I do," says Larry, leaning over to whisper in my ear. "Courage."

"You're better at this than I am." I mean it. I can feel the acid spill of jealousy eating me.

"I'm not better, I'm different. You're his mother. I'm his father."

"I'm the heavy. I think you've got the better job."

"I think we just walked into San Francisco's Times Square," says Larry. "What a scene!"

"Garden of Eden. Live. Adam and Eve Totally Nude. Hey, everybody! I'm totally nude!" Adam is reading the neon marquees. "Tunnel of Love. Big Al's. Totally Nude Girls on Stage. Man-Woman Love Act. Playland at North Beach. New Hong Kong Noodle Company. The Condor Presents Carol Doda Topless Love Act . . . Can we go in the noodle company? Do you think they make the noodles there or just sell them there?"

San Francisco's Broadway is a sexy Disneyland, an oxymoronic playground for good dirty fun over which a three-story vertical paper-doll image of Carol Doda presides, looking prim as Snow White in a scant black bikini. Blinking neon nipples ride her cleavage like maraschino cherries on vanilla scoops. Beneath her amused, affectionate eye, men in business suits, like naughty dwarfs, misbehave.

A noisy crowd of women carrying placards is gathered in front of the Condor. "Don't do it, Carol. Don't be a boob!" they chant. Some of the signs they carry bear the single word "WHO."

"Who is WHO?" I wonder aloud into the round face of a baby riding in a canvas sling on her mother's back. The baby smiles merrily at me between apple-red cheeks.

"Who is this Carol person?" Larry asks no one in particular.

"Mommy, what's a boob?" Adam asks.

The woman with the baby on her back turns to answer. Suddenly, as if I had needed just one more to go "gin," I am face to face with a queen.

A frenzy of long, springy black hair, parted in the middle and tucked in a temporary truce behind each ear, makes a triangle of her head. Small, fierce, deeply set blue eyes peer out from deep sockets beneath finely arched brows. Her nose is high, bony and bent, like a hawk's. The face of a sphinx, or a witch.

Beads, belts, scarfs . . . she looks as if she has put on everything in her closet in a hurry, but the overall effect seems intentional—stylish.

"WHO is a women's feminist organization," she says. I had not expected an aristocratic English accent. "Double-U, aich, O," she explains. "That's an acronym standing for whores, housewives, and others. It's a good name, don't you think?" Then, without waiting for a reply, she addresses herself to Larry. "The Carol person is Carol Doda." She pauses for a moment, waiting for some sign of recognition to congeal on our faces, and seeing none, asks, "Are you new in town?" She flashes a huge smile, far wider and warmer than the limits of her thin, pursed lips had implied. She is either ugly or beautiful. I can't decide which.

"Yes, we are," I offer. "We just got here yesterday."

"That explains it," she shrugs. "Carol Doda is San Francisco's most famous topless dancer. She works in this night club right here, the Condor."

"What's a Condor?" Adam asks.

"It's a large bird, a kind of vulture, actually, I think," the woman answers.

"It really means 'the golden cunt' in French," Larry whispers in my ear. *Le con d'or.*

"But what's this demonstration about?" I ask.

"Bosoms," the woman answers. "Carol Doda's bosoms, to be precise. By the way, my name is Sara. Sara Urquhart Duskin." She extends her hand, first to me to shake, then to Larry.

"I'm Mary-Lou Weisman. This is Larry."

"Hi," says Larry. "Any relation to Sir Thomas Urquhart?"

"Yes, as a matter of fact!" Sara grins. "How on earth do you know about him?"

"I was a comparative literature major at college."

"Who is he?" I ask.

"A seventeenth-century Scotsman who translated the works of Rabelais," Larry answers. "Right?"

"You're right!" Sara shakes her head.

"Then you're Scottish. I thought from your accent you were English."

"My parents sent me to England to be educated."

"Isn't Scotland where the Loch Ness monster lives?" Adam asks.

"Yes, that's right. In fact, there's an old ruin called Urquhart Castle that overlooks Loch Ness, where Nessie is supposed to be living."

"Have you ever seen the monster?"

"No. I've never spent any time at Urquhart Castle. The roof's been off for hundreds of years. I lived in a castle called Craigston. Sorry"—she offers her hand to Adam—"no monsters at Craigston. Just my mother, my father and Nanny. What's your name?"

"That's all right," says Adam. "I'm too old to believe in them, anyway. I'm Adam, and this is my brother Peter, but we call him Pete or Petie most of the time, except when we're pissed off." I wince a *pro forma* maternal wince, but my heart's not in it. The name of today's game seems to be dickies, boobs and cunt, so what's a little "pissed off" among strangers?

"What your baby's name?" Peter asks. "Is he a boy?"

"No, she's a girl. Ceres Ann Urquhart Duskin," says Sara, doing a quick turn, rotating herself and spinning the baby in and out and then back in view, as if she were wedged in a revolving door. "Ceres, say hello to Adam and Peter." There is a silence while we all wait for what is clearly not going to happen. Ceres can't be more than two or three months old. She just blinks. "If she says hello, I'll be very surprised," says Sara. "She's only three months old, and she hasn't said anything yet. Still, you never can tell. One of these days it's going to happen."

There is another pause. "Nope," Sara announces. "today is not the day."

"That's okay," says Peter.

"I never heard of someone named Ceres before," says Adam. "It sounds like cereal."

"It does, rather, doesn't it?" Sara bites her top lip thoughtfully. "She's named after the ancient Roman goddess of agriculture," she adds, as if that somehow explained everything.

"I have a silly name too," Peter offers.

"Are you permitted to tell it to me or is it meant to be a secret?"

"It's private, but it's not secret."

"May I try to guess it? It's so much more fun that way. Is it Parsley?"

"Nope." Pete giggles.

"Is it Zephyr?"

"Nope."

"How about Parsnip?"

"I don't think you're going to get it," Peter advises. "I think you'd better give up."

"All right. I'll give up, but just in the interest of saving time, you understand. I might have gotten it if I'd kept on at it."

"It's Fudgetickle Entworth LaRue."

"I rather like it," Sara says. "Fudgetickle Entworth LaRue." She pronounces each syllable slowly and solemnly, as if she were presenting him at court. "It's a splendid name. It has everything—humor, substance, good breeding—and, of course, fudge. That's probably the most important part. I love fudge. Whose wheelchair is this?"

Nobody answers.

"Well," chirps Sara, undaunted, "since it doesn't seem to be anybody's wheelchair and since I could be anybody, then it might be mine, and if it were mine, then it's not likely that anybody would object to my sitting down in it for a while, is it? It's time for me to feed Ceres." She turns her back on Larry and talks to him over her shoulder. "I wonder if you'd be good enough to hold on to Ceres for a minute whilst I sit down. Then I'll take her from you." Sara scooches down, palms braced on her knees, while Larry lifts Ceres up and out of the sling.

"Wow! She's heavy!" says Larry. "Heavier than she looks."

"She's built like her father. Solid."

"Is your husband here?" Larry asks, taking Ceres over his shoulder and snuggling his head against the side of her cheek.

"No. Alvin doesn't usually come to feminist events. He says that worrying about women's rights in 1972 is like wondering if your children have had a good breakfast on the *Titanic*. He's out hunting with the rest of the men."

"Hunting?"

Sara laughs. "It's my personal theory—it's not too popular with some of my feminist friends—that, generally speaking, men are the hunters and women are the gatherers. The women mind the base, tend the children and perform the civilized versions of tasks like gathering firewood, picking berries and digging for roots and tubers whilst the men hunt.

"Of course, there's no big game anymore, so they hunt in the economic or political arena looking to make a killing."

"Do you mean that you think those qualities are inborn?"

"Yes, more or less. But there's a catch. Women have varying amounts of the hunter in them, and men have varying amounts of the gatherer in them. I have a bit too much of the hunter in me for comfort."

"Boy, I hope your neolithic update is wrong. It sounds like a bum rap to me."

"It is. It's impossible. To simultaneously want to bear and rear children and to want to make a killing does not make for happiness," Sara concludes, opening her blouse and reaching for Ceres. "It requires stamina and a great sense of humor."

"Cosmic," I agree, watching Sara's dour, craggy profile soften to a madonna's. I have decided. She is sometimes ugly and sometimes beautiful.

"What does your husband do?" Larry asks.

"Up until a few months ago he was in the garment business—the Alvin Duskin Company. Now he works on his political projects."

"Such as?"

"At the moment there are two he cares about especially—Public Interest Communications, it's called—and he wants to write an initiative to force a vote on nuclear power here in California."

"What's Public Interest Communications?" Larry asks.

"It has to do with buying media time for interest groups who can't normally afford it." Sara pauses for a moment. "Do you remember the Mexican who hijacked an airplane a few weeks ago?"

"Yes."

"Do you remember what his demand was?" But she doesn't wait for an answer. "All he wanted was five minutes of television time to tell the country about the plight of the migrant farmer. That's the problem in a nutshell. This is a country where access to the media is crucial. If minorities don't get it, they're going to take it. Right now, Alvin and some of his friends are working on helping prison workers organize a union. They have this crazy idea that they can get the Playboy Foundation to fund the project, or at least to give the prisoners free ad space in the magazine."

"Crazy like a fox," Larry comments. *"Playboy* is the most popular magazine in the prisons. Alvin sounds like an interesting man; I'd like to meet him."

"Well, then," says Sara, "why don't you come to dinner—all of you—tonight. But I warn you. He'll get you involved in PIC or the antinuclear initiative—or both. He's very charismatic." Sara touches the tip of her index finger to her nipple, releasing Ceres' hold on her breast, and shifts her to the other side.

"What about Carol's boobs?" I am reminded. "What are all these people waiting for?"

"Any minute now Carol Doda will appear, topless, in

front of the Condor," Sara explains. "Her bosoms are famous, you know. They're huge. She's had them pumped full of silicone so they just stick straight out, defying gravity. It must be dangerous. I hate to think what might happen if some of that silicone broke loose and began to travel through her bloodstream. But that's not the issue. What's supposed to happen today is that Carol is going to make an impression of her bosoms in the freshly poured concrete in front of the Condor. It's a publicity stunt, to drum up business."

"Kind of like Grauman's Chinese Theater?" I ask.

"Exactly, only San Francisco style."

"It's funny."

"It 'tis funny," Sara agrees.

"It wouldn't be funny back East. Eastern feminists would stone her."

"Not if they recognized the considerable amount of Carol Doda that dwells in every one of them." Sara takes Ceres from her breast and closes her blouse.

"That's where a sense of humor comes in handy." I take Ceres from Sara's arms and lower her legs into the backpack.

"That's what I love about WHO," says Sara, shrugging the backpack into place and straightening up. "Look!" Sara points toward the Condor. "See? See those two heavyset men in the white short-sleeved shirts? They're the bouncers. And there's Carol!"

There she is. Barbi Doll on a half shell. Her hay-straight, white blond hair is distributed in two lacquered hanks in front of each shoulder. Her boobs survive the build-up. They are sturdy, amazing, death-defying.

But it is her skin, oh my God, her skin! So white, milky-white, poreless, opaque, exquisitely tender. I can see the blue network of her veins. She stands, flanked by two goons, stripped to the waist, wearing nothing but black stretch slacks and high-heeled mules. She is Joan of Arc, transcendent, facing the fire. She is, head shaven, disgraced, a Jewish maiden turned German SS slut. I have to remind myself that she does this for a living, gladly. This is Carol Doda, working her way to Las Vegas, smiling and waving to the crowd.

"Don't do it, Carol," the women yell, waving their signs. "Don't be a boob!"

"After all this waiting," says Sara, "they'd be furious if she didn't go through with it!"

Sure enough. Held aloft by the two men, one supporting her beneath the shoulders, the other holding her thighs, slowly, slowly they lower them into position like torpedoes, aiming them at the sidewalk below. She disappears horizontally, to the mixed reviews of catcalls and cheers.

"I'm curious to see what kind of a mark two bosoms make," Sara remarks after the crowd has begun to disperse, "aren't you?"

"Probably two identical craters," says Larry, helping Peter into the wheelchair and following Sara's lead.

"Probably like two stainless-steel ice cream cones with cherries on top turned upside down," says Adam.

"Carol didn't make much of an impression at all!" All I can see is a Rorschach of two identical amoeboid, tacky-textured splotches on the otherwise smoothly poured concrete.

"I think the concrete must have hardened up too much beforehand," says Sara.

"Mommy?" Pete says. "What are those marks on the sidewalk?"

"What do they look like to you?"

"Like mouse ears. They look like Mickey Mouse's ears."

"The Duskins have exactly fifteen steps, not counting the landing, leading to their front door," says Larry softly behind gritted teeth, "and that gallant little bugger is going to insist upon climbing up them by himself. Hey, Pete," he calls out, kneeling and outstretching his arms, "hop in! I'll give you a free ride!"

"I can walk up the steps by myself," says Peter, stopping to examine the flight of stairs, which must seem to him no less formidable than a ziggurat.

We are doing this all wrong, I mourn to myself; we are

doing this all wrong. If we could keep it up, maybe we could get away with it, but we won't be able to keep it up. We won't be able to get away with saying that the wheelchair is for resting and everybody needs a rest; and that you just hop a ride on Daddy when the going gets rough and people put ziggurats in your path, and Daddy will always be there, big enough and strong enough, no matter how big you get—we never say strong—to distract you with free rides. And we won't be able to get away with throwing the scissors in the trash because—bad scissors—they must have gotten dull or bent because Petie cannot make them open and close and he could just last week. The family motto—act as if nothing is happening—but how else to act, what else to say, when what is happening is too terrible for words, unspeakable.

But what, I ask myself—just as the grandfather in *Peter and the Wolf* ominously warns Peter in the record—"What if a wolf should come out of the forest? What would you do then?" Except that in our case it's not a matter of the what-to-do-should-the-wolf-come-out-of-the-forest; he's out.

"I want to climb the stairs by myself."

Larry shrugs an "I give up, let him do it." We wait, and watch.

Peter sees that there is no banister. He will not be able to use his usual technique, pulling himself up the stairs with his arms, his body following, so slowly and reluctantly that I feel my own arms tremble with effort, and my own torso turn and strain, and feel the paint-chipped black iron banister cold and scabby against my cheek.

Peter sees that he will have to crawl up, the less agonizing, but more humiliating alternative. Babies crawl. We wait, and watch.

He places his hands, palms down, on the second step. Pushing down on his palms he fools gravity by relieving enough pressure from the lower part of his body so that he can lift his own feet. The right knee tests the air, slowly, as if it were dense, and then kneels on the first step. The left knee does the same; a little more quickly. I breathe. There are fourteen more. We wait for him at the bottom so he can wait for us at the top. Time hovers over his effort, thick, suffocating.

At last he is on all fours on the landing, like a child playing doggie. He looks around for a prop. A wicker laundry basket filled with shoes—too low, flexible, uncertain. The door. It will have to be the door. He crawls toward it, first placing his left hand, palm down, on the little wooden lip of the threshold extending out from under. His right hand follows, flattening itself against the panel, his fingers crawling like the itsy bitsy spider up the water spout. They inch their way upward, dragging the palm behind them, until Peter senses he has achieved ideal leverage. Then his left hand abandons the threshold and takes its place on the door. The knees unbend slowly, one after the other, until his bowed torso is stretched taut, suspended between two points: the palms of his hands and the bottoms of his toes. The fingers of both hands crawl upward just a little bit more, and Peter is standing. We made it.

Adam and Larry and I begin to mount the steps, not too quickly, that would betoken impatience; not too slowly, that might suggest a pitying sympathy; so we mount the steps at an ordinary pace, a pace that does not call attention to itself, and act as if nothing is happening.

"Lift me up, Daddy, so I can push the buzzer."

See? A perfectly normal seven-year-old who cannot reach the doorbell.

"I walked all the way up the stairs," Peter boasts to Sara as soon as she opens the door. "I'm strong."

"You're better than strong," says Sara, kneeling to give him a hug. I watch her put her arms about Peter, and then tighten her grip on him when he threatens to topple over. "You're better than strong; you're tough."

"Do you want me to break the spaghetti in half or shall I just drop it in unbroken? That might make it easier to handle with chopsticks." A male voice comes from the kitchen, followed closely by the man who must be Alvin.

"Hello," he smiles from the kitchen doorway and walks toward us, extending his hand. "Sara told me about you. I'm glad you could come. I'm Alvin."

The first thing I notice is the lisp—not the ordinary slurpy, sloppy sort, but a soft, satiny one that seems to come from both sides of his mouth, from tiny gaps where the top and bottom teeth don't quite meet, except for the upper and lower canines, which make contact at their points. His smile is generous and self-satisfied; disarming and demonic.

He is a big man, and well-built. The muscles and tendons of his forearms seem to lie on top of the skin. His hands are large and weighty, his fingers long and thick.

Handsome isn't the word, I think, as I check out his thinning brown hair, the puffy lids over pale-blue eyes, the long nose. Sexy. The word is sexy.

The dinner table looks like the bric-a-brac table at a garage sale. Crystal goblets are lined up with five-and-dime glasses. Spode nestles uneasily with Mexican earthenware dishes. The forks are a spiky clot of stainless steel and silver. Six sets of chopsticks protrude from a plastic weaning cup. It is an eclectic rubble, the distressing evidence of momentary whims, doomed fresh starts, contradictory lifestyles, and oppressive heirlooms. It looks to me as if the owner had been trying to unburden her cluttered soul in one paroxysm of "Harry, we've got to get rid of this crap" and was planning, tomorrow, having already saved enough register tapes, to buy an eight-piece starter set of ironstone, Dusty Rose pattern, at the supermarket. Ceres, the centerpiece, presides over it all in an infant seat, like a damp Irish drunk in a deck chair.

"What are the chopsticks for?" Pete asks.

"The spaghetti," says Sara. "Look, I'll show you how. Pay attention. First, you take one chopstick in each fist and stick them straight down in the pasta." She demonstrates like a picador running at a bull. "Then you wrap your hands around both sticks together, like this, and then you start to turn them around slowly, until you've got a good-sized glob, like this. Then," she says, very slowly, very thoughtfully, having just attempted unsuccessfully to bring it to her mouth, "you simply lay your head down on the table, like this, curl your lower lip under the rim of the plate, like this, and just push it in. Very restful."

"That's messy," says Peter.

"Would you prefer a fork?"

"Yes."

"Me, too, please," says Adam.

"Perhaps you're right," Sara allows. "I just thought this might be fun."

"If Sara were called upon to reinvent the wheel, she'd start by experimenting with a cube, just on the off chance that, over the eons, someone might have overlooked a good thing." Alvin flashes his impressive dental line-up once again.

"Be grateful I haven't questioned eating off plates yet. Which plate would you like, Adam? Pick your favorite. You, too, Pete."

"I want the orange one with the black swirls," says Adam.

"You picked my favorite!" says Sara. "I got that one at a flea market in Sausalito for a nickel. It's all right, though. I like this one next best." She reaches into the middle of the pile. "I swiped it from home."

"Sara tells me that you spent some time at Esalen," Alvin begins, leaning back in his chair, looking at Larry. "Why did you do that?"

"Someone besides me was bound to ask me that question sooner or later," Larry says with a smile. "I've been trying to account to myself for it over the last few weeks, even before we left Esalen, and I haven't come up with anything but embarrassing answers."

"Such as . . . ?"

"I think I went because I was bored—a kind of premature mid-life crisis. No, worse than bored; disheartened. I couldn't generate any enthusiasm for what I was doing. Besides, something had happened that caused me to doubt all my preconceptions and made me want to re-examine my life."

"Yes." Alvin nods, indicating that he knows.

"But that sounds suspiciously high-minded, doesn't it?" Larry sits straight up in his chair. "Cut it down to size, and what you've got is a thirty-two-year-old man who fell for the most foolish hustle of all—the search for happiness."

"And did you find it?"

"What?"

"Happiness."

"No, just the search. Esalen is the travel agent for optimism. I bought a fistful of tickets, but they all turned out to be round trips. Perhaps I'm not a good traveler. I can't, or perhaps I don't want to—that's what they'd say at Esalen—overcome my essential, cautious nature.

"But I sometimes wonder if what I wasn't participating in was some heartfelt but ultimately doomed effort to cure humankind of the human condition. I'll probably never know. Meanwhile, I'm stuck somewhere between Pangloss and Job. In a few months we'll be going back to Connecticut to cultivate our garden and, undoubtedly, to bitch some more."

"How about you, Mary-Lou?" Sara twirls her spaghetti with her right hand while nursing Ceres at her breast. "What was it like for you at Esalen?"

"I never fit in. Not from the first day. It was like being in the Garden of Eden."

"That sounds rather nice . . ."

"Except that I was the snake."

"Do you have a couple of aspirin?" Larry turns and asks Alvin.

Alvin gets up from his chair and heads toward the kitchen.

"Bring me a diaper whilst you're up, please, Alvin," says Sara.

"Anybody want a beer?" I hear Alvin call.

"I'll take one, thanks," Larry calls back.

I can hear the beer cans hit against the inside of the kitchen garbage can.

"Alvin!" Sara scolds. "I bet you threw the beer cans in with the egg shells I'm saving to feed the chickens. He always does that," she tattles, like a married woman in love.

"Do you have chickens here in the middle of the city?" Adam asks.

"They're in the garden, just out there." Sara points toward the back of the house. "I'll introduce you to them after dinner if you like."

"How do you know about chickens? Did you live on a farm?" Peter asks.

"Not exactly. Craigston is a castle, but my mother kept chickens so I learned about them from her, and also about pigs and cows from the farmers. I used to love to slop the pigs and milk the cows with the farmers' kids. It was always so much warmer at the farmers' houses."

"Was it cold in the castle?" Peter pronounces it like Sara, "cah-sle," and smiles at the sound of himself.

"Every time I went to bed I had to carry firewood with me up two hundred cold stone steps to my bedroom. It's very cold in castles. On the other hand, they're very good for roller-skating. Lots of long corridors."

"And she gave it all up, the baps, the scones, the steamed treacle pudding, and all the other Scottish delicacies that, once eaten, remain in your body indefinitely, to marry a Jewish garment manufacturer. Here's the diaper"—Alvin drops it over Sara's shoulder—"and here's the beer."

"Thanks." Larry puts the aspirin in his mouth and swallows some beer.

"How long are you planning to stay in San Francisco?" Alvin sits back down at the table.

"A few months. We have an appointment to keep in England in August. We'll head home from there."

"What are you going to be doing while you're here?"

"I'm not sure. Nothing at the moment. This is what I

claim I've been waiting for—nothing to do. Now we'll see. I've got my doubts. I seem to be flunking moments of truth lately. There are plenty of books I've been saving to read, but I've got a feeling I'm going to get restless. I'm even beginning to miss practicing law."

"Well, if you get restless, you could work at Public Interest Communications. We'll be approaching some foundations for money in the next couple of months for the prison-reform project, and it would help if you'd come along with me. We could use someone who looks and acts halfway respectable." Alvin grits his teeth, smiles and looks devilish.

"If you and Larry work together, you'll have to buy yourself a proper button-down shirt instead of always wearing that workshirt, and put your jacket on a hanger instead of dropping it on the floor." Sara buttons up her blouse and puts Ceres over her shoulder.

"The prison project sounds interesting; I'd like to hear more about it," says Larry in a tone of voice I haven't heard for months—Horatio Alger–eager. "When do I start?"

I laugh out loud.

"What's so funny?" Larry challenges, knowing damn well.

"You!" I can't stop laughing. "You sound so . . . so Eastern."

"And what's the matter with that?"

"Nothing!" I'm still laughing. "I love it! I've missed it. I've actually missed you being an uptight asshole."

"Do you have any plans for yourself whilst you're here?" Sara asks me.

"I'm not sure. Betty Fuller said she could arrange for me to lead some groups. I might take her up on her offer."

"Well, if you have nothing better to do, I'd love to involve you in my women's bookstore and coffee-shop project. I've got the concept; now I'm looking for the proper location. It would be a place where mothers could bring their children during the day and stay themselves to talk or read. I'm also considering selling clothing wholesale at the same location if I can work out a deal with the Alvin Duskin Company. With your help, we might get it started in a couple of months!"

"God! Where do you get all the energy? When Adam was three months old, it was all I could do to put dinner on the table."

"Sara's very fierce about doing something besides what she's doing," says Alvin. "She always has a scheme."

"It's not for pleasure; it's just how I am. I can't stop planning."

"I'll be happy to help you. I could use a scheme myself."

"Damn it!" Suddenly Larry clamps his hand to his head. Above his clenched fingers his brow is gray and folded with pain. I expect him to scream, but instead he speaks with a whispered, last bit of control.

"I'm sorry, folks. I hate to break this up, but I've got to go home. I've got a terrible headache."

"Maybe some more aspirin?" Sara asks, heading for the kitchen.

"No thanks. I've been taking them every few hours for days. They don't seem to help much. Maybe if I lie down for a while . . . I feel as if I've got a lead balloon in my head."

"You'd better see a doctor right away," I say in response to the concern which implodes in my chest, all the while wondering why I haven't paid any attention before.

Larry reaches in his pocket for the car keys.

"I'll drive," I offer, putting out my hand.

"You're scared of the hills," he says, but he hands me the keys.

"Let's go!" I call, leaning over to pick up Pete and hoisting him onto my hip.

"Strong lady," says Alvin.

"Careful on the steps!" Sara calls after me. "There are fifteen, not counting the landing."

"You can take your goddamn marriage contract and shove it up your ass!" I sob. Oh shit! I hate it when I cry. I always cry when I fight. Oh shit!

"Look," says Larry in his now-let's-be-reasonable voice, "I

know we didn't have a contract, but we did have an understanding, a conventional understanding that I would go to work and earn the money, and you would take care of the house and the kids. I don't know what you're grousing about. We both have a lot of free time now. I have no job. You have hardly any housework. I'm free to help Alvin out with the prison project. You're free to hang out with Sara and lead groups, and if you don't want to have to be here when the kids get home from school, you can hire a baby-sitter. Besides, sometimes I'll be home, so you won't even need a sitter. I like to be with the kids. You know that." Very pleased with himself, the very soul of rationality, Larry rests his case. "So, for Chrissakes, pick up the phone, get yourself a baby-sitter, and you can go out, too!"

"Why don't *you* pick up the fucking phone and get *yourself* a baby-sitter?" I sob with rage.

"Because that's not my job!" Larry slams his fist into his palm. "Don't you understand?"

"No. I don't understand. I don't see any difference between us at all. We are both unemployed. We are both parents of these two children. We both know how to cook and clean. We both have things to do outside the house, so I don't understand why I am always responsible for calling the baby-sitter."

"I'll tell you why. Because I worked for seven years to make the money that's paying for this year."

"I hate you!" I cry, leaning forward, hurling the words at him with the spit that flies from my mouth. I have lost all dignity. I might as well be nine years old, yelling, over the hedge that divides our properties, at my anti-Semitic best friend, Pam Clifford, "The Jews did not kill Jesus!" but wondering if they did.

"I'm going to get a Kleenex," I whimper, retreating to the bathroom, tripping on the rug.

"Jesus Christ," I hear Larry hiss with frustration. "You're giving me another goddamn headache."

I slam the bathroom door. There is no Kleenex. I take a

swipe at the toilet paper, bang the toilet seat shut, sit down and sob. Following some unarticulated command to "calm down," I gulp the anger into my stomach and feel sick. I can hear the children in the kitchen.

"I can't get the refrigerator door open, Adam. It's stuck."

"Okay, I'll get it. What do you want in here?"

"An orange, but I'll get it. You just hold the door open. I can get it by myself."

"How long are you going to run away for?" I hear Adam ask.

"I don't know for sure. Maybe forever."

"Then you should take some Devil Dogs."

"Mom only lets us take one," says Peter. "She says it's crap."

"You doo-doo! If you're running away from home, you might as well take as many as you want. You won't be here for Mom to yell at you."

"Okay."

"See?" says Adam. "This is how it's done. First, you put all your supplies in the middle of this bandanna."

I sit on the toilet, my arms wrapped around my legs, feeling the bristle of my knees under my chin, while love and enchantment calm my heart.

"Then you gather up the corners, smiggle them into a knot, and then you tie the bundle onto the end of this stick."

There is a knock on the bathroom door. "Mary-Lou!" Larry calls. "I think you'd better come out. There's some funny business going on out here." His voice is full of love. "Come on." The only demand I have left is that he must open the door. He does.

"Pete is planning to run away from home," Larry reports, helping me gently off the toilet seat. "I've been listening to them from the living room. They're adorable."

"I know. I've been listening from the bathroom. I felt as if I were some wise old queen of the wood sprites, perched on a mushroom deep in the enchanted forest, eavesdropping on their souls. They're wonderful."

"Then you put the stick over your shoulder. There! Now you're all ready to run away. You look perfect! Here, you'd better take a dime in case you need to call home."

"I can't reach the phone in the phone booths."

"That's no problem. Just ask someone to help you."

"We can't let him go, Larry."

"Yes we can. Running away from home is one of the important things kids do. I ran away from home; didn't you?"

"No, but I thought about it. I thought about it a lot. Usually in the bathroom. I understand that it would be good for Pete, but I think it's too risky. I'm scared that something will happen to him. Christ, Larry, the elevator door could close on him. He can barely make it through in time."

"We've got to take that chance. We'll watch from the window. Let's go. Come on. If anything goes wrong, we'll just rush right down." We hear the elevator door slam. I hear my heart soar.

"Peter Benjamin Weisman has run away from home," Adam announces as we emerge from the bathroom. "He's really pissed off at you guys for arguing."

"You were really nice to help him," I say, giving Adam a hug and a kiss. "You're a terrific brother."

"I was scared you'd be angry with me for letting him go. I know it's dangerous, but he wanted to do it so much, I just couldn't—"

"That's okay. You did the right thing," says Larry.

"I was going to go with him, but then I figured it was the sort of thing a person had to do alone."

"I think you were right about that, too, Addie," I say.

"Meanwhile, he could kill himself." Adam shrugs, California style.

"Right again, kiddo," says Larry. "That's why we're watching from the window. So far, he hasn't even gotten out of the building."

"Something has probably gone wrong already!" I cry. "He could have fallen down inside the elevator. Maybe he fell down in the foyer." I have no courage for this.

"Let's wait just a few more minutes. We've got to try to let him have a normal experience."

"But he's not a normal kid, Larry. We can't pretend he's a normal kid!"

"He is, too, normal," says Adam. "He just can't walk so good."

"So well," I say reflexively.

"So well," Adam grouches.

"All right," says Larry, suddenly reaching a limit that I did not observe him approaching, "I'm going down. It's been at least five minutes. He should be outdoors by now."

"No!" I hear myself cry. "Don't go! Let Adam go. Is that okay with you, Addie?"

"Sure. We're buddy boys."

"Hurry up, Ad," Larry urges, spanking him on the ass like a football coach. "You know," he says as we watch Adam run down the hall, his Big Sur knife tied around his thigh with a string of rawhide, "you are wonderfully sensitive. Your instincts are so sound."

"See?" I explain, trying to prolong the sweet feeling his compliment has given me. "If Pete is in trouble, then he's going to feel particularly failed and humiliated if you or I rescue him. But if Adam helps him, he'll still have his dignity."

"I understand that. I just don't think I would have thought of it."

"Well, you were right about letting Pete run away in the first place. I'm not sure I would have had the nerve to let that happen."

"Well, then, with your sensitivity and my nerve, we make one whole person, one whole marriage, don't we?" Larry wraps an arm around my shoulders and jostles me toward reconciliation.

"I guess we do." I hang my head.

"Do we have a truce, then?" Larry is wide-eyed, smiling, expectant.

"We have a truce. And we do. Except that I know it's only

temporary. Hey, what happened at the doctor's?" I ask.

"He gave me a complete neurological work-up and found nothing."

"Great. Are they considering surgical removal of your head?"

"He gave me some codeine and told me to come back next week."

"Does the codeine help?"

"A little, but it nauseates me. He gave me something for that, too."

The apartment door swings open to reveal Adam, arms stretched wide.

"Ta-dum!" he announces. "Pete's decided he's run away from home long enough!"

Peter enters, beaming, swaying gently from side to side.

"Oh thank God you're back at last!" I cry, rushing toward him. "I was afraid you'd never come back, that you'd left us forever!" I overact. "Your father and I were worried sick!"

"You were?" Peter asks, clearly pleased. "I wasn't gone *that* long. You don't have to kiss me so much."

"Maybe it didn't seem long to you, but it seemed like forever to us. I'm so glad that Adam persuaded you to come home."

"He didn't persuade me, exactly." Peter will not be conned.

"You must have had a terrific adventure," says Larry. "Will you tell us about it?"

"Well, first I walked all the way down the hall to the elevator. Then I stood up on my tiptoes and pushed the button that has the arrow pointing down. And *then*"—the excitement mounts in his voice—"then the elevator came and the doors opened and I told myself 'Hurry up, Pete,' and I hurried up and I got through just in time! And then I rode all the way down with myself in the elevator. Then, when the elevator landed and the doors opened, I told myself 'Hurry up' again and I got through again just in time! Then I was in the lobby."

"And *then* what?" Larry asks.

"And then I couldn't get the door to the outside open. It's too heavy."

A trap door opens in my chest, and I fall through. I set up the pratfalls, and then do my own emotional stunt work.

"So then what did you do?" Larry does have more nerve.

"So then I decided I would just wait awhile and a friend would come and open the door."

"And did a friend come?"

"Nope."

"So then what did you do?"

"So by then I was getting hungry. I tried to untie the bandanna, but the knot was too tight . . ."

"So then what happened?"

"Then Adam came and saved me."

"So he opened the door for you?" Larry asks.

"No. He opened the bandanna. Then we ate all the Devil Dogs. And after that we ate the orange."

"So what made you decide to come home?" Larry asks. "It sounds as if things were going pretty smoothly. Let me guess. I bet you missed us."

"Nope."

"You ran out of Devil Dogs?"

"Nope. I wet my pants," says Peter.

"It must have been all the excitement," says Adam, who must have heard that once before and just now made the expression his own.

"Well," I laugh, "I remember wetting my pants once when I was a little girl."

"How little were you?" Pete asks.

"Well, I was older than you are. Let's see . . . you're seven. I was nine, I think. Lots of older people wet their pants," I say so confidently, that even I have a picture in my mind of crowds of adults writhing, lurching around on Van Ness Avenue, cross-legged, hands cupped against their crotches, their mouths wide open like in *Guernica,* their eyes round with panic. "Mommy, I gotta go! I gotta go to the baf-froom!"

"Lots of them?" Pete asks, touchingly insistent on the truth.

"Well, maybe not lots. I do tend to exaggerate. But quite a few. A surprising number."

"What do they do when they wet their pants?"

"They usually are smart enough to do exactly what you did. They come home and change their pants," I say, tugging gently down on the elastic waist of Peter's corduroy trousers. I don't buy the ones with zippers and snaps anymore. Peter can't do the snaps.

"Just a minute!" Larry intervenes brusquely. "Before you do anything to that kid, he's got to be punished. A person who runs away from home has to be punished. And that's final."

"What are you going to do to my child?" I plead, tugging at Larry's trousers.

"Sorry, lady, I'm going to beat him up." Larry swoops down, picks up Peter, and sits him on the kitchen counter. "Okay, kiddo. This is it!"

Larry adjusts Peter's chin so that his head is perfectly straight, facing forward. He places his left hand, palm open, just below Pete's ear. Then he raises his right hand and brings it down diagonally, swiftly. His open hand misses Peter's cheek by a fraction and slaps, instead, with a stinging smack, against the palm of his left hand, waiting beside Pete's ear. I am holding my breath.

"Do it again, Daddy," Petie giggles. "Do it again."

Larry does it again.

"Again, Daddy."

And again.

"Jesus Christ, do you believe this kid!" I hear a catch in Larry's voice as he throws his arms around Pete and holds him close. "You're an amazing kid, Pete; you're a champ." Larry is as proud as if Pete had just pitched a Little League no-hitter. "Okay, soggybottom," he says, lowering Pete to the floor, "go change your pants. Adam will help you." He gives Pete a playful little slap on the fanny.

"I can't get over it," Larry says, shaking his head back and forth in a soliloquy of wonder and unashamed feeling. "He knew to the marrow of his bones that I would never hurt him. He trusted me completely. Like William Tell's son, he didn't even flinch." There are tears in Larry's eyes.

"Chin . . . up! Chin . . . up! Everybody loves a happy face. Wear . . . it! Share . . . it! You can brighten up the darkest place . . ." We are sitting at dinner. Peter is singing to Larry, whose aching head is plunged into his hands. His palms exert a special focused pressure on his temples, as if he could twist the pain away.

"Spar . . . kle! Twin . . . kle! Let a little sunshine in. You'll be happy-hearted, if you just get started, up with your chinny chin chin . . . up! Up with your chinny chin chin." Pete's sweet voice, reedy, meandering unselfconsciously from key to key, reveals only the most tantalizing hints of melody, although scrupulously insistent that the word "chin" always be at least a couple of tones lower than the word "up." He carries the tune of consolation.

"Does your head feel better now, Daddy?"

Larry lifts his head to smile. "Maybe a little. Thanks, Pete. That's a terrific song. Where did you learn it?"

"I think it's a pukey song," says Adam.

"Where did you learn that word?" I demand in accordance with some ancient maternal oral tradition.

"From you," chirps Adam, delighted to have caught a parent in his parent trap.

"I learned it at the Sunshine School. Our teacher, Miss Orne, makes us sing it every morning. You don't have to pretend you feel better if you don't, Daddy. It never makes me feel any better. It thought it might work for grownups."

"I'm going to lie down for a while. Maybe I can sleep it off, okay? I'm sorry to leave in the middle of dinner. I seem to be doing that a lot lately."

I watch him leave the table, his back bent, his head low,

his arms limp. He places one foot in front of the other with the precision of an old man.

"Larry, phone the doctor."

"Look, we've been through this before," he calls back, his voice weary yet hostile. "Will you get it through your head that I do not wish to call the doctor! He doesn't know what is the matter with me, never mind what to do about it. Besides, I have an appointment to have some tests in the hospital. Christ, I hope they will show something, anything. A brain tumor would be welcome news. I hardly care."

"Please, I don't want to annoy you, but will you please call the doctor, if not for your sake, then for mine." I wonder why it is that whenever I hear myself say phrases like "If not for your sake, then for mine," I imagine that I am holding someone else's script, suddenly reading some other actor's lines—is it Arlene Dahl, Deborah Kerr, or maybe Susan Hayward? Did I spend too many Saturday matinées preening in front of the tempting, fantastic emotional plumage of the fifties? Is MGM producing, directing and collecting royalties on my innermost feelings?

"Just let me get some sleep, will you? I appreciate that you're worried about me," he says with courteous sweetness, "but the best thing I can do right now is get some rest. Good night."

"Good night." I lower my head and pick up my fork.

"Mommy's pissed," says Adam as soon as he hears the bedroom door shut.

"I just wish he'd see the doctor more often, complain louder, make a fuss, insist."

"You're the mommy," says Peter. "It's your job to take care of people."

"I'm *your* mommy, but I'm not Daddy's mommy. It's not my job to tell Daddy what to do."

"Why don't we call Grandma Rosie and get her to tell Daddy what to do?" says Adam.

"That's not a bad idea, Addie. We'll tell his mommy on him!" And we all have a good laugh.

"I'm magic," Peter announces between mouthfuls.

"What kind of magic?" I ask.

"I can make people sick," Peter brags uncharacteristically, with the kind of ferocity that betokens hurt. Suddenly I am a mother animal, instinctive, wary.

"Who have you made sick lately?" I smile up from my fork, keeping it light.

"My teacher at school, Miss Orne. It worked, too. We had a substitute teacher today."

"What worked? What's your magic technique?"

"Voodoo. Adam showed me how. I stuck a needle into my stuffed hippo's stomach last night and today Miss Orne didn't come to school."

"What did Miss Orne do to deserve a needle in her stomach?" I see Peter's eyes flinch with injury.

"When I fell off my chair because I was fooling around, and it served me right for fooling around, she wouldn't help me get up and she wouldn't let anybody else help me get up either." He is fighting tears.

"You mean she just left you on the floor?"

Peter nods.

"For how long?"

"Till the end of the class."

"Oh, Fudgetickle, you must have felt so sad!"

"Yes," he says.

I hug him tight.

"Your teacher is an asshole," says Adam.

"Don't use that word," I cuff, but not too hard, because he used it for love. "Do you know Miss Orne's first name?" Then I remember that Peter sometimes gets mixed up about what's first and what's middle—he is always sure about the last. "You know, her first name, like Mary-Lou, or Peter or Adam."

"Alice," he says. "I think Alice."

I reach for the phone book.

"Let's see . . . There are lots of Alans. Oh, damn . . . there are one, two, three Alices, not to mention four just plain

A's—she's probably the A-type ... Eight-two-six, nine, three, six, four. It's ringing," I report, my hand over the mouthpiece. I am full of heat, steamy fury and nervous glee.

"Hello? I'm phoning to speak with a Miss Alice Orne who teaches at the Sunshine School . . ."

"Yes, this is she."

"This is Mary-Lou Weisman, Peter Weisman's mother."

"Oh, yes," she says.

"I'm sorry to have to call you at home, especially when you're ill, but Peter has just told me a very disturbing story about something that went on in your classroom, and I'd like to discuss it with you now if you are able."

"Certainly," she says. "I'm feeling much better, thank you; it was just a mild stomach ache."

"Well, first of all, I'd like you to tell me whether or not it is true that you left Peter on the floor after he was fooling around and fell out of his seat."

"That is correct," she says.

"Would you please tell me how on earth you justify your behavior?"

"I am not in the habit of justifying my behavior, Mrs. Weisman, but I'll be happy to tell you why. I did it to teach Peter a much-needed lesson. I warned him several times to stop wiggling in his seat, but he refused to obey.

"I trust he will be more obedient in the future, although I am afraid that Peter has a serious problem accepting authority. You know, Mrs. Weisman, the best way to deal with handicapped children is to treat them like normal children. You mustn't feel sorry for them, or they'll take advantage of you, just like normal youngsters," she advises me sternly, leaving me momentarily winded with outrage and staggered by her blunt, bestial logic.

I want to kill her . . .

"In my opinion, Miss Orne, you have no right to be teaching children, handicapped or otherwise. I intend to air this matter with your principal. I hope you'll be there."

"I'll be happy to be there, Mrs. Weisman. I am sure that

Miss Quint agrees with me that we cannot have children disrupting the classroom with disobedience and fresh talk. Goodbye, Mrs. Weisman." The phone clicks, diminishing the conflict to an insulting, linear buzz.

. . . and tear her limb from limb . . .

"Christ! What a horrible woman!" I snarl, replacing the receiver.

. . . and leave her for the buzzards . . .

"You were great, Mommy!" Adam applauds. "You really got pissed off."

"I wonder what she meant by 'fresh talk,' " I muse, returning to the table. "Did you say something fresh to Miss Orne, Peter? Not that I would blame you," I add for encouragement.

"Promise not to get mad if I tell you?"

"I promise. I need to know the whole story if I'm going to talk with the principal."

"Well," Peter says slowly to his plate, "I didn't say anything fresh out loud then, but, second period, when she asked me to come to the blackboard and write the date and the weather, I wrote *'Fuck you.'* I couldn't help it, Mommy, it wasn't my fault," Pete hurries on, "it was an accident; I didn't mean to," he says, fixing his face with a look of sly consternation while he rummages through his brain for a suitably adult-sounding excuse. "Something must have come over me," he concludes darkly with a sigh, satisfied that he has come up with the right one, until he dares to look up from his plate into our laughing faces.

"I'm glad to be alive," says Larry, smiling up at me from the hospital bed, the top of his head helmeted in a mummy's cap of white gauze and adhesive tape. His smile is so sweet, so serene.

"Doesn't your head hurt?"

"Believe it or not," says Larry with great spunk, "this is the first time in four months that I haven't had a headache."

"Oh, Larry! I'm so happy. You look wonderful. I was so

scared. The doctors were really afraid that they wouldn't get you into the operating room on time, before the blood clot—well, I don't know . . . before it, I guess, sort of blew up. Once you were in the operating room they told me and Sara and Alvin that there was nothing more to worry about. It's a simple operation. The ancient Egyptians performed it all the time."

"Shut up and come on and sit down next to me. Forget the ancient Egyptians."

"Are you sure I won't jostle you?"

"I think I want to be jostled," Larry answers with a funny leer I can't quite recognize. I sit down gingerly on the side of the bed. Larry immediately puts his hand in my crotch.

"Jeezus Christ! What are you doing?" Someone in me knows exactly what he's doing, but most of me doesn't believe her.

"Let's make love," says Larry tenderly, shifting himself to his side and moving backwards, making more room on the bed. His head is slightly raised from the pillow in the effort.

"Larry! Stop it! Something terrible could happen! You could start bleeding!"

"I feel fine. Nothing hurts. I feel terrific. See how terrific I feel?" Larry reaches for my hand and presses my palm against the starchy white folds of the bedsheet, which sheathe a full erection.

"You're crazy! For God's sake, you're crazy!"

"Let's make love," says Larry plainly, surely and quite sanely.

"I'm afraid to. I'm afraid for you. You were just operated on a few hours ago. It must be dangerous. The strain. The increased heartbeat. We can't do it."

I know I am right, and yet I feel no conviction, and therefore no resistance. "We can't do it, Larry," I repeat. "The nurse might come in."

"I knew I could convince you. Now get up and go lean that chair against the door. Prop it up just under the door-knob." I obey.

"Okay," I say, "but only on one condition."

"What's that?"

"That you lie flat on your back and I'll do all the moving."

"I agree, on one condition."

"What's that?"

"That you take all of your clothes off. I don't want to feel like a two-bit lay."

"What if someone comes in and here I am fumbling into my underpants in the special care unit? They'll arrest me, for Chrissakes!"

"No one is going to come. No one is even going to try."

"How do you know?" I ask, already stupid enough to believe he might actually have an answer.

"I just know," he says, as if he did.

I let go of everything sensible and undress.

"Now get under the covers."

I do.

Larry is still on his side. He puts his arms around me and holds me tight against his angel robe. We kiss, softly, tentatively. Sweetness flows. I fill with life and intent. "Remember. Lie still on your back."

I brace my arms and slowly, carefully maneuver myself on top of him, feeling the tip of his penis trace a line across my belly. Larry sighs. I listen one last time for the tiny shrieks of white-soled rubber heels moving hastily down highly waxed linoleum corridors, and lower my hips to take him in. I slip my hands, palms up, under his buttocks. A sigh catches in his throat. I move up and down slowly, lasciviously, showing him every glistening crevice, imagining his pleasure and guiding him to it, deep and slow, deep and slow, until rhythm turns to passion and I lose command.

"I love you!" Larry cries as we stiffen, then shudder in each other's arms. My face feels the tears on his cheeks.

"Oh, thank God, thank God." I reach between my legs to feel the welcome wetness.

"See?" says Larry, recovered from the passion. "I told you

nobody would come!" And we giggle wildly, out of control, stuffing edges of sheet into our mouths to muffle the sounds, for all of those dry mean years.

"When we get to the beach, let's bury Pete," Adam calls over his shoulder as he struggles to push the wheelchair along the sandy pathway leading from the parking lot to Pfeiffer Beach.

That small person inside me, the bleeder, lurches and sinks to her knees as if shot in the gut. "Sure," I call ahead. "If he wants to."

"It's hard to believe that in a week the four of you will be in England. We're going to miss you." Sara bends toward me as we walk, pausing momentarily to readjust Ceres, who is riding on her back. "Now that it's almost upon you, how are you feeling about the spirit doctor?"

"Detached, oddly detached. I'm interested in going through with it. In fact, I don't think I could *not* go through with it, but not because I have any hope."

"You can't really afford to have any," says Sara, "but you never can tell . . ."

"That's true, but there's more to it than that. Something has happened. I can't imagine Peter being well anymore. I used to be able to do that, up to a few weeks ago, but now I can't. Peter and his disease have disappeared into each other. Now the sick Peter is the real Peter. A well Peter would be an impostor."

"Shit!" Adam mutters, expertly levering out the wheels by jumping onto the chrome bars which project alongside the rear wheels.

"Hang on a sec, Addie," I respond, called into action. "If I pull from the front while you push from the back, I bet we can get Pete onto the beach. Then we'll bury him." There, now, I think as I lope toward the children, that wasn't so hard, Mary-Lou. Bury Peter. Why not? Where's your sense of humor?

"Ready, set, go!" Adam announces as I grab the tubing

beneath the armrests, lift up the front of the chair and begin to walk backwards in a crouch toward the open beach.

"We're a pushmi-pullyu!" I smile up through the strain at Peter. "Remember the animal in *Doctor Dolittle* that was the same in front as in the back?" Lowering my head, I watch out for rocks or furrows in the patch of sand that moves continuously forward between my legs.

"You're a strong mommy," says Pete, filling me with strength.

"You're a tough kid," I answer, giving him all I've got.

"Turn around, Mommy, we're here!" Adam's voice trails off with a squeak of excitement.

I turn in time to see a great white wave explode into spume as it hurls itself slowly through the vault of a huge archway of rock—living land cut off from the California coast by earthquake or glacier, or trickled away by the patient severance of the tides; lopped off and distanced, standing far from shore, proud and lonely as the Arc de Triomphe at dawn, an orphaned leviathan wading in the cold, chaotic sea. A moon, cool and sly and insubstantial as magic, hangs in the daytime sky.

"Wow!" says Adam, in a rare moment of childish wonder.

"Well, what do you think?" Sara asks Peter.

"Good," says Pete.

"That's all you can say?" I prompt. I want Peter to be happy, to sound happy, to yell with glee like a happy child.

"What about you, Mary-Lou? Do you like it? Isn't it the most beautiful beach you've ever seen?" Sara reaches her arms out wide and white against the sand bars that curve and stretch like languid nudes lounging on their sides at the water's edge. The waves lap unevenly against the sand, leaving an imprint like a lion's paw.

"It's beautiful," I say, feeling the blood swell and thrash in my chest, tasting brine in the back of my mouth. "And scary."

"How did the rock get way out there?" Adam asks.

"That's an interesting question. I was just thinking about

that myself. Maybe it happened all at once, broken away by an earthquake. Or maybe it could have happened during the Ice Age, slowly, by water erosion."

"Or maybe he was never attached; maybe he was always out there all alone. Maybe he was born that way," says Peter.

"Let's bury Petie now," says Adam. "I'll start digging the hole so that you'll have something to put him down in. The sides of the hole will help support him."

"I can sit up by myself."

"Adam just means that you'll be more comfortable if you start out sitting in a hole."

"I'll help," says Sara, struggling out of her backpack. "Pete, you keep an eye on Ceres, just in case she decides to eat sand or go swimming."

I kneel in the sand, ready to dig, my body poised, trying to remember how. The feel of the sand pressed into my knees, the exquisite bite of each disparate crystalline grain, jogs my memory: the feel of braids swinging against my collarbone; the lunge, scoop and pull of my shoulders; the rasp of wet sand against my finger pads, hoarding itself luxuriantly under my nails; the mountain of excavated sand growing and snug between my legs.

"Do you want to use my shovel?" Adam asks.

"No thanks. Don't trust shovels, never did. The metal shovels we used to use always bent. Then they rusted. Then they broke. Then we cried. By hand is better."

"This shovel is plastic," says Adam.

"That's worse. They don't even bend; they just break," I prattle on, feeling those braids swing, those arms scoop, those fingers burn. I hear myself slurp my saliva back into my mouth like a child.

"Do you think it needs to be bigger, Adam? What do you think, Sara?"

I pause, brush my hands together and cock my head. "Maybe just a little bit more on your side, Adam. That's great. This is going to be a terrific hole, don't you think, guys?"

"Sara! She's eating sand. Ceres just ate a great big mouthful. I think she likes it!" Peter smiles down on Ceres like a proud mama.

We all stop to watch Ceres' face change from grin to howl behind the tiny hand, as plump as a starfish, pressed against her mouth, awaiting the verdict on the new taste sensation.

"Spit it out! Go pleh-pleh-pleh!" Sara demonstrates, jiggling up and down like a marionette, spitting away imaginary sand with gusto.

Ceres just sits there and cries with outrage.

"Oh, it's horrible, isn't it Ceres! Oh, you poor thing, it's awful," Sara croons, rushing toward Ceres. "We'll fix it. Mommy's going to fix it. Come." And she grabs Ceres from the sand and carries her, red and rigid, to the water's edge and bathes her face gently. "It's getting better now. See? It's getting better," she says soothingly. "It's feeling better and better, and soon it will be gone." Ceres gives one final whimper against the cure and is comforted.

"Can I get buried now?" Peter begs.

I straighten up, place my hands on my hips, take a deep breath and close my eyes, searching inside me for center.

Peter examines the hole from his wheelchair.

"Do you think you can lift me up and then way down?" Pete is learning how to worry.

"Of course I can. Remember me? I used to be the strongest mommy on the Eastern seaboard; now I'm the strongest mommy on the West Coast," I brag, wondering.

"Can you pick me like a petunia?" Peter's lips smile around our private language.

"Like a petunia." I straighten up, place my hands on my hips, curl my toes into the sand and take one more deep breath before reaching to slide one hand beneath his thighs, burrowing the backs of my fingers as deep as possible into the vinyl seat until I am free on the other side; the other hand I move easily across his back and grip under his arm.

"You're magic, Pete," I whisper into his ear with a kiss. "Make yourself light."

"I don't know how to do that."

"Just think 'marshmallows' and 'feathers' and 'ping-pong balls.' "

"Marshmallows, feathers, ping-pong balls. Marshmallows, feathers, ping-pong balls," Peter chants, squeezing his eyes closed, tilting his wishful, furrowed face to the sky.

As your child grows heavier and more helpless, the necessary lifting becomes too much of a strain for the mother . . . The words of Public Affairs Pamphlet No. 271 drag across my brain, trailing failure. I bend my knees and bounce, testing them as if they were springs. I take another deep breath, feel the wind in my face and the sand solid beneath my feet, and lift Peter quickly and smoothly and close against my body so I feel his weight as if it were my own. Slowly, carefully I walk toward the hole.

"We did it, Pete! You *are* magic." I smile as I lower him, with confident strain, into the sandy hole, marbelized with streaks of seaweed, twinkling with mica.

"Did I really make myself lighter, Mommy? Did I really? You're not just pretending?" Peter is scrupulous.

"I can't be absolutely, positively sure, but I think so. In fact, I'm almost positive you felt lighter." I am not absolutely sure myself that I am just pretending.

"Okay, ladies and gentlemen, the kid's ready to be buried!" I call. "Adam, why don't you and Ceres bury Pockie, and Sara and I will go for a short walk together." Suddenly I can't bear to witness the sight of speckles of black grit covering his luminescent skin. "Just make sure that you protect his face and especially his eyes from the sand," I call cheerfully over my shoulder even as I shiver at the thought.

I can tell by the way she says "Mary-Lou" as soon as our backs are turned on the children and we begin to walk down the beach that Sara has been rehearsing. "I hope you don't mind . . . we really don't know each other that well . . ."

I begin to interrupt with a gesture of "Oh no, that's not true," but I give it up in deference to her candor. Besides, she's right. We don't know each other that well.

We have walked up and down the sun-spangled streets of North Beach together nearly every day for months, hunting and gathering, she with Ceres riding on her back, I pushing Pete. Like sharks who must keep swimming or die, we cut through the crowded streets in constant pursuit of anything—the perfect coffee bean, some sourdough bread, the place that makes homemade pasta; or if we get through the gathering list, we hunt for the right location for Sara's coffee shop, bookstore, wholesale clothing outlet and child-care center, a place where she can sit down, take Ceres off her back and share the burdens of motherhood. We never find the right location, but at least we keep moving, keeping each other company, talking each other through yet another day, the way a cop talks a suicide off a window ledge. But we don't know each other that well. We teeter on the cusp of intimacy. We do not know each other so well that we admit our desperation. We call it shopping.

"Don't say 'no.' It's true. We're friends as much because of our husbands and the fact that we're both tied down by children, as by our own free choice."

"Those are good reasons, too, aren't they?"

"I think so," Sara smiles, "especially when you add to that the fact that we're both foreigners and we're both lonely. I was so glad you showed up when you did. I was happy for your company."

"I've been grateful for your company, too. It might have been a bleak few months for me without you. I don't know what I'm going to do without you when I get home. My only real friend, Glenda, has moved to Concord, Massachusetts."

Home. All I have to do is say the word and my chest fills with a panic that must be like drowning. Home is where we have to go now. Home is where the music stops. Home is where Mother lifts the phonograph needle off the record at my birthday party and there is no place for me to sit down.

"That's what I want to talk to you about, if I may . . ."

"Sure."

"I'm worried about you. The more I observe you and Peter and Larry and Adam, the more worried I get about all of you, but you in particular. I see you getting angrier and angrier with Larry, more and more distant from Adam, and sinking deeper and deeper into Peter."

"I know. It's true. I don't know how to stop it. It's something that's just happening."

"After all, Adam is going to grow up and get more and more involved with friends and with school. Larry, no matter how much he involves himself with Peter and you, still has his law practice. But what will you be left with when this is all over besides a lot of bitterness, anger and sorrow?"

"I don't know. It worries me, too."

"Well, it *should.*" Sara switches from the future tense to the feminist inspirational. "You've got to take care of yourself. You're going to need something of your own to hang on to. Have you considered getting some kind of job when you get home?"

"I might try to get a job working for a newspaper in Westport."

"You mean the one you told me about, the paper you were involved in just before you came to California?"

"Oh, no. *The Turtle* only lasted a couple of months, just until the black kids were accepted into the Westport schools. It was a one-issue paper. Someone wrote me that some of the same people who backed *The Turtle* are setting up a weekly regional paper to be called *Fairpress.*"

"I'm really happy to know you're considering that." Sara takes my hand and gives it a squeeze. "You need to care about something outside of Peter. He's going to get weaker and weaker and more and more dependent upon you. He's going to pull you under, bit by bit. It's going to take a lot of effort to resist. It's hard enough for determined women to have lives outside of their children's. It's going to be especially difficult for you. Anyhow"—she smiles one of her big, wide well-that's-that grins—"I'm glad to learn that you're not planning to be a living sacrifice. Come on!" She begins to run along the beach, pulling me after her.

But I hold back, resisting her momentum. "Sara? What if it turns out that my life *is* a sacrifice? What if it turns out that that's what loving Peter and caring for Peter requires?"

The only answer is the crying in the wind. "Shhh!" I hiss, holding up my hand. "I think I hear Peter."

We freeze.

"I don't hear anything," says Sara. "You're imagining it."

"No, I'm sure. Something's wrong. Let's hurry back. Run near the water, it's faster," I yell over my shoulder. My legs stretch, my heels pock the wet sand. Cold water lashes my ankles; the wind parts across my face; my hair flies. In the distance I see Adam kneeling, his back to me, hurriedly unburying Peter, whose wailing grows louder.

"What's the matter?" I say, coming to a stop in front of the mound on which sits Peter's head, like Brave Mr. Buckingham. Without his body, he looks normal.

"Pete doesn't like being buried," Adam explains. "I'm unburying you as fast as I can," he says into Peter's wet and weeping face. "You don't have to scream your ass off like that!"

"I thought you wanted to be buried, Pierre Ginzberg La-Farge," I say, dropping to my knees, helping Adam scoop, playing it straight.

"I did," Pete snuffles. "But now I hate it."

"Well, then, we'll unbury you!" I smile, adopting a tone of logical levity. "Some people like to be buried, some people don't. You never know which kind you are until you try."

"I couldn't move!" Peter's voice is full of horror. I watch him move his arms and legs slowly, as fast as he can, as each limb is freed of its burden of sand. "I hate it!"

I curl up alongside him in the hole, put my arms around him and touch as much of him with me as I can.

"It was awful not to be able to move. I felt bad," he offers.

"I'm sorry you had such a bad feeling."

"The feeling is getting better now," he reports.

"I'm glad." I squeeze him with one final hug, meant to wring the last drops of sorrow from us. "Since we're all so sandy, why don't we go for a swim before we head back to San Fran?"

"Whoa!" says Sara as she tucks Ceres in her backback, guiding first one pudgy leg and then the other into the canvas openings. "We didn't bring our suits, and besides, this isn't really a swimming beach. It's too cold and dangerous. Sometimes people surf here in wet suits, but you really have to know what you're doing."

"Well, then, we'll go wading. Okay, guys?"

"Can I go too?" Pete implores from his hole.

"Of course you can. I'll pick you," I yell over the muted roar as another wave breaks, slow motion, through those colossal legs, froth trailing like bubbly banners in the air.

"Like a petunia?"

"Just like."

"Do you think you can pick me from way down?"

"Don't worry, I know I can."

I straighten up, place my hands on my hips and take a deep breath, swelling my belly outward. Then I test my knees, bouncing downward to a crouch. I sense Sara move in and stand behind me. I burrow my right hand in the sand, palm up, and watch my forearm disappear beneath Pete's thighs. I tunnel the other behind his back and test his weight by rocking him slightly to and fro. I rid my fingers of sandy grains by brushing them gently against his thighs, and tighten my grip. "Marshmallows," I murmur between gritted teeth. "Here we go!"

One adrenal surge of the will, slipped past a drugged defense, and I am standing with Peter in my arms. With one hand gripping his bottom, I use the other to guide his legs around my waist and to reach his arms around my neck, pausing long enough for him to join his hands to keep them up by lacing his fingers.

"Ready, Adam? Ready, Sara? Let's go, guys!" I whoop,

setting out across the beach with Pete in my arms, gravid with his weight, feeling the sun heat my cheeks and the sand grow colder and more solid beneath my feet as we walk into the water.

"Is the tide going in or out?" Sara calls. "I'm never sure."

"I'm not sure myself," I call back. "We won't go out too far."

"Let's go out as far as the lonely monster," says Peter. I can feel his excitement as a barely perceptible twitch of tendons around my waist, and the frail flutter of his fingers laced in my curls.

The waves slouch toward us, flowing through my legs, cold, bracing and familiar, mixing with the brine of my blood, tempting me forward. My clothes feel like the wind; my mouth tastes like salt.

Like a mountaineer or a suicide, I succumb to the urge to risk it all. Each wave that breaks behind my knees seems to stop, reverse direction and go berserk, streaking madly between my legs, defying nature, confounding perception, flowing backwards out to sea. I stand, looking down, locked in terror, watching my eyes deceive me, like a passenger in a stalled railroad car being passed by another.

I am mesmerized, dizzy, swaying precariously; my toes grip for dear life at the eroding sand which seems to break away and speed between my feet like a ribbon of highway reeled in. Who is moving? Who is standing still? The horizon tilts. Sky slips between my legs. Oh God help me I am falling!

Like a ballerina tumbling from a pirouette, desperately, instinctively I look up and around, searching for something fixed and far to spot, to keep me standing. I find the rock.

"Which one's the doctor, Chapman or Lang?" Larry asks, glancing up from his travel guide. "I keep getting them mixed up."

"I'm not sure either. I think Chapman's the doctor, and Lang's the fireman."

We are sitting in the waiting room of Chapman-Lang's office in Aylesbury, England. I don't know what I was expecting, but I know this wasn't it—a modern one-story brick office building. I hadn't pictured an interior so bland, so beige, so unchallenging to the eye, so aseptic to the imagination.

Graceless wooden chairs line the walls. The two wood-grained, rectangular Formica tables are heaped with journals and magazines. The requisite waiting-room rubber plant, with its fat flipper leaves, is lashed to a stake of bark-covered log. Rubber plants are peculiar to doctors' offices, the way jade figurines are to New York hotel lobbies.

In this setting we must look like a family awaiting its six-month dental checkup instead of a miracle. What decorative style was I expecting, I wonder—Victorian paranormal? Plum velvet drapes? Fringed lampshades? A floating table?

"Come to think of it, it's Lang. I'm positive the doctor is Lang. I think."

"They're *your* spooks," says Larry. "The very least you could do is remember which is which."

An elderly lady gets up from her chair and approaches the nurse's desk tentatively, holding her purse up in front of her chest, like a modest maiden stepping out of her bath. "Could I please make an appointment to see Mr. Lang in the autumn?"

"Mr. Lang doesn't make any appointments in the early autumn," the nurse replies, wetting her thumb against a tiny round sponge that sits, soggy and willing, in a tiny round white ceramic bowl, and turning the pages of the large appointment book open before her on the desk. "His hayfever bothers him too much. How about late November? Will that do?"

"What's the doctor going to do to me?" Peter asks from his perch on Larry's lap.

"He's going to examine you and see if he thinks there is anything he can do to help your muscle problem." I never say "muscular dystrophy," except when I have to; for instance, if a nurse needs to know "for Doctor's records." Then I can't say he's got a muscle problem. Then I have to say "muscular dystrophy," no matter how much it hurts me.

Muscular dystrophy is a poster child, a telethon, a dread disease I've hardly even heard of. Every time I say it, I learn for the first time that Peter is dying.

"Hey, Pocket," says Larry, giving Pete a little jostle on his lap, "hey, Flush Water Tinkle Pop McGee, how'd you like to go to visit this place after we get done with the doctor?" Larry holds the guidebook open for Peter.

"How do I know if I want to go if I've never been?" Peter responds with not a hint of sarcasm.

"I guess you're right. When are you going to know, do you think?" Larry asks with deference.

"When I get there," says Peter.

"Spoken like a true here-and-now Californian," says Adam. Adam is seated next to Larry, trying to get a Slinky to walk from one knee to the other by gently elevating one bent leg.

"And as for you, doofus, what do you think? You always have an opinion." Larry hands the book to Adam. "Read it to Mom and Peter."

" 'Woburn Abbey,' " Adam reads aloud, " 'has been the ancestral home of the Dukes of Bedford for over three hundred years and is one of England's leading stately homes. Following the present Duke's decision to live abroad, the house is lived in by his eldest son, the Marquess of Tavistock and his family.

" 'Woburn has one of the greatest private collections of works of art in the world. The State Apartments have the superb elegance of the seventeenth and eighteenth centuries and are hung with paintings by many of the world's great masters, including Claude, Gainsborough, Frans Hals . . .'

"I think I've got an opinion," Adam interrupts himself. "It sucks."

"Not so fast, hot shot," says Larry. "Keep reading."

" 'Woburn Abbey also includes the largest drive-through

Safari Park in Great Britain. On your way round you can see majestic lions and tigers, graceful antelopes and zebras, giraffes, camels and brown bears right through to lumbering rhinos and hippos and playful monkeys. There is also a self-service snack bar, supplemented by a pub called the Duke's Head and by kiosks at various points on the grounds selling ice cream, soft drinks and candy.' "

"It sounds good, Adam," says Pete. "Let's go."

"I thought you only knew if you wanted to go somewhere after you got there," Larry teases.

"That's before he heard about the ice cream," says Adam.

"It was the candy," says Peter, who needs to be precise.

"Mr. Lang will see you now." The starched white nurse's cap, riding lightly on top of steel-gray curls, tilts gently in our direction, like a schooner dipping in the waves. Dumbly, in response only to the authority of her voice and through no will of my own, I get up from my chair.

"You stay here, Adam," I say, touching him lightly on the shoulder. I look to Larry and see that he is already standing at attention, with Peter in his arms. Larry's face is playing it straight.

We move through the waiting room, past the nurse's desk, past the distinguished-looking man in the tweed jacket with the leather elbow patches, reading the *Manchester Guardian;* the same man who had said earlier, "Believe it or not, I was completely blind two years ago. As blind as a bat." It is difficult to doubt the integrity of an Englishman in leather elbow patches.

The formerly blind man winks and mouths "Good luck" as we walk by. I try to smile back, but my face won't work. We approach the closed door at the end of the hall.

Larry hikes Pete farther up in his arms. I raise my hand and prepare to rap my knuckles lightly on the door when I see the knob turn and the door begin to open inward.

Light from the corridor spills into the darkened office. From within, ruby-red wall lights beam like jeweled eyes.

"Enter, please." The voice coming from behind the door has the thin, reedy timbre of very old age. Yet a certain tension gives its accent the strangulated, histrionic quality common to British character actors. I look down at the doorknob, my eyes straining to adjust to the dim light. The hand on the doorknob is very well-kept and young. "Please enter."

We file all the way in and turn slightly to the right, awaiting the man who is stepping out from behind the closing door.

"Good afternoon, I am Mr. Lang," he says, removing his hand from the knob and turning away from the meticulously closed door to face us. It does not matter that my jaw drops, that my hand moves instinctively to my open mouth to forbid some startled cry. As if caught in an agonizing blaze of light, Mr. Lang, his eyes clenched shut, smiles genteelly in our direction through the tortured, furrowed topography of his face.

"Mrs. Weisman," he says, bowing slightly at the waist and extending his hand to me. We shake.

"Mr. Weisman," he says, bowing slightly, his hands at his sides. If his eyes are shut, how can he know not to shake hands with Larry because Larry's holding Pete, I wonder, looking at him, noticing how his trim body is tensed into an old man's round-shouldered stoop, how he cocks his head to listen, how the heavy black three-piece suit, watch fob and graying Vandyke suggest photos of Freud.

"And you must be Peter Weisman," he says, patting Peter right on the top of his head. He's peeking. He's got to be peeking.

Emboldened, I scooch down a little and look him dead in the clenched eyes. He doesn't seem to be peeking. I back off. What if he can . . . ?

"Now, Mr. Weisman, if you will be good enough to place Peter on the examining table right over there, I'll do my very best to help you."

My eyes, now accustomed to the amber darkness, seek out

amid the shadowy furnishings of his office and find what must be an antique examining table of dark-stained wood and wine-colored leather.

"Don't be frightened, young man," Mr. Lang says to Peter, who listens calmly. "I promise you that nothing I do to you will hurt you. Do you understand?"

"I understand. I believe you," says Pete.

"Good," says Mr. Lang, helping Pete to stretch out on his back on the table. "I'm just going to take off your shoes." He moves unfailingly toward the double-knotted bows on the tops of Pete's high-top brown Oxfords, and begins to untie. "Mother's got you all tied up here, doesn't she, young man? Now, let me see, it's America you come from, isn't it?" Mr. Lang turns away from Peter to address Larry.

"Yes," Larry answers, "from Connecticut, near New York."

"Delightful. Delightful. Have you by any chance had the opportunity to pay a call at Woburn Abbey?" A little paranormal small talk.

"No," I answer, "but we're thinking of taking the children there later this afternoon."

"The Duchess is a lovely woman—full of dash and dazzle. It's such an enormous household to run, such a terrible financial drain, but you never catch her complaining. I suppose sooner or later the Duke of Bedford will have to give it up, turn it over to the National Trust. That will be a shame." Mr. Lang's speech is high-pitched and slow. "Yes . . . yes . . ."—his voice cracks—"just set the stable boy's leg last week."

"We're going to have ice cream and candy," Peter offers.

"How very lucky you are. Give the Duchess my best regards," says Mr. Lang and turns to hand me the first shoe. "Would you take this, please, Mrs. Weisman?"

My mouth and my palm open flat. He places the shoe neatly in the middle of my hand and turns back to Peter.

What if he can . . . ?

"Yes, yes"—his voice cracks with effort—"I first met the

Duke and Duchess what you might call 'professionally' when I set the stable boy's broken leg." Mr. Lang forces out a wheezy laugh that makes me want to yell, "Come on! Come off it!" But I don't. I put out my other hand to receive the other shoe, which he holds out to me, his flamboyantly blind face straining intently into mine.

I dare to steal a glance at Larry, who shoots one furtively back at me. We both act as if we were being watched.

What if he can . . . ?

"Would you like me to take Peter's clothes off?" I say what I say to the pediatrician.

"No thank you, Mrs. Weisman, that won't be necessary," says Mr. Lang, flexing his fingers and then swooping them down and up into a pair of imaginary rubber surgical gloves. Elbows bent, he rotates his hands outward, and holding them in front of his face like votive offerings, he turns toward Peter.

"Now I shall operate on Peter's spirit body and attempt to produce a corresponding effect in his physical body." His eyes remain clamped shut; his mouth slightly open, expectant. He holds his head forward a bit, cocked, tense, as if straining to hear a conversation in the next room. He passes his gloved hands, palms down, over the lower part of Peter's body, traveling from waist to knees, to feet and back again, slowly, about two inches above his skin. Peter lies quietly.

The gentle stroking motion ends abruptly with the thrust of Mr. Lang's arms, the flex of his wrist, and the stretch of his palm as it reaches upward in the air. "Basil," he says curtly.

For a moment the hand remains stiff and arched in that position and then he snaps his fingers. "Basil!" When did he take his gloves off? You can't snap your fingers with rubber gloves on.

Then his fingers close around an invisible object invisibly delivered, and he turns back into a silhouette to face Peter. With his imaginary scalpel he cuts a fine line of an incision down both of Peter's legs, from the tops of his thighs to the tops of his toes, about two inches above his skin. "I am increasing the circulation to the lower extremities," he explains.

Quickly, the hand shoots out again. The fingers snap. Impatience. Another snap. A pause. His fingers close. With his imaginary scissors, he snips the veins and arteries in Peter's legs, about two inches above the skin.

What if he can . . . ?

Clutching Peter's shoes, I stand and watch the needles threaded, the stitches sewn, and the handings and takings of surgery, until the last pantomime suture is pantomime-clipped, and the gloves—they are back again—ripped off with the studied abandon of macho medics, or a crazy man playing doctor.

But what if he can . . . ?

Mr. Lang reaches toward Peter to help him into a seated position. This is the time and the place for a miracle.

A child, limbs rounded and glowing, illuminated by the golden dust of downy hairs, leans the flats of his hands against the examining table, springs nimbly to the floor, spreads his arms wide, proclaiming himself like an eagle in flight, and runs across the floor into my open arms. "Mommy!"

I look at Peter sitting on the examining table, thin arms turned outward, the flats of his palms constantly renegotiating the delicate balance of his slumped torso, while his legs hang heavy and lifeless, bringing him down. "Mommy!" he calls. "Pick me, Mommy, pick me like a petunia."

He can't. Of course he can't.

"Now," says Mr. Lang as I give Peter his shoes to hold and pick him up in my arms, "I know it may not seem as if Peter has been through any sort of tiring experience, but let me assure you he has. I recommend that he rest for at least two hours this afternoon." He begins to move us toward the door, grinning and nodding and trying to see through his own face.

He can't. Of course he can't.

"Would you mind telling me whether or not you think you've been able to do anything for Peter's condition?" I ask, although I know the jig is up.

"Of course I can't be certain," he says cheerily, "but I did operate in such a way as to increase the circulation of blood into the legs. That should help to relieve his condition." He opens the door.

"Shall we make another appointment with you?" I am unable to stop.

"Certainly, if you like."

"When do you suggest?"

"Perhaps in a year," he answers nonchalantly.

"Fine, we'll do that," I say, having no intention whatsoever.

"Make an appointment with my nurse," he says as he closes the door.

Of course he can't, you stupid asshole, I harangue myself as the door clicks shut. The man is crazy. Almost as crazy as you are.

"Just do me one favor," says Larry as we rush past the nurse's desk and out into the street. "Could we make an exception to our usual manner of dealing with things and not talk about this?"

"For how long?" I ask.

"I'm not sure," he answers. "Maybe forever."

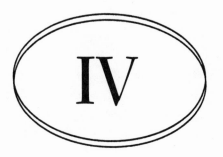

"Which one of you guys remembers what our house looks like," Larry teases, making a left turn onto Greenwood Lane.

"I do! I do!" Peter calls from the back of the car. "I do! It's the one with the swimming pool in the backyard that you can't see from the front."

I do. I do. It's the dark-green shingled ranch house with the concrete ramp in the front. Home. Sorrow tugs at my heart like a child on a sleeve.

"Welcome to the Holy Ghost Hospital for the Terminally Ill," reads the sign on the lawn of a hospital I used to drive by on my way to Brandeis. I remember wincing each time I saw it, fearing that the patients would, one day, get a look at the front of the sign and learn their doom. And I wonder if he knows.

The house slides into view. A red Volkswagen is parked in the driveway. "GMPC" reads the license plate. Ever since the divorce, Mother has been threatening to have it changed to GMP ("Who the hell wants any part of *his* name"), but each time she is deterred by the thirty-dollar fee.

"It looks as if Mother is here to greet us."

Larry's knuckles whiten as he grips the steering wheel tighter. "I wish she'd hold off long enough for us to get settled."

"Me, too. It's hard enough to be back."

"Actually, it's really very sweet of her, I suppose," says Larry, loosening his grip. "I shouldn't be so nasty. She means well. Hey, guys!" he calls over his shoulder. "Grandma is here to welcome us home."

"Shit!" says Adam. "I just want to see my room, and then I want to go swimming."

"Since Mother's parked in the turnaround, why don't you park the car right in front of the ramp. That'll make it easier to get Peter out," I say.

Mother hasn't noticed us yet. I can see her profile in the car window. She is knitting.

"It looks more like a stakeout than a welcome," Larry quips, guiding the car to a stop.

"Welcome home! Welcome home! Ga-reetings! Ga-reetings! Ga-reetings!" Mother warbles, rushing toward us, flapping her arms in imaginary ecstatic hugs.

"Hi, Mother."

"I've been waiting for two hours," she scolds, placing her hands on her hips. "You said you'd arrive by lunchtime. It's three o'clock. I've been sitting here for two hours, starving to death."

"I didn't know you were planning to meet us. You should have left and gotten something to eat."

"And take the chance of not being here to welcome you when you arrived? No siree. You should know your mother better than that by now."

"You bet your sa-weet ass you should," Larry mutters as he turns off the ignition and pulls up the brake, nudging me in the ribs. I turn toward him fast enough to see him curl his lip, hitch it over his teeth, Bogart style, and lisp, "Welcome home, sweetheart."

While Larry escapes to unpack the trunk, Mother stands up against the car door, holding me hostage, lecturing to me through the half-opened window. "Nobody likes to be kept waiting, Mary-Lou. It's a form of rejection. You know how sensitive I am to rejection."

"Don't bother to fight," Daddy advises as he leaves the house for the last time with his suitcase and his Strad, while Mother is having her hair done. "With her, all victories are Pyrrhic."

"I'm sorry, Mother."

"You haven't even asked me how I am."

"How are you?"

"I'm fine, thank you." She nods.

"And how are my two da-arling grandchildren?" she smiles into the back seat. "Skin and bones . . . both of them. Thin as rails." She shakes her head in vigorous dismay. "Let's see what I have in here for you!" Now she makes her voice secretive, tense with untold delights while she rummages in her black lizard pocketbook.

"Here it is!" She waves a stick of Juicy Fruit on high. She folds it carefully, tears it in half and hands one half to each child. They reach for the gum. She does not let go of her end. They tug. She hangs on.

"What do you say?" she prompts, her eyes expectant, encouraging.

"I love Juicy Fruit," says Peter. "I'm glad you brought it for me."

She still hangs on.

Pete's face, once lit by his wet, pink smile, all gleamy with anticipation, darkens with bewilderment.

"What do you say?" she repeats to Adam.

"Thank you," says Adam, and the gum is released.

"Thank you?" Peter tries.

"Now there," says Mother. "It's not so difficult to be nice, is it?" And Peter gets his gum.

"Come on!" yells Larry, breaking the spell. "Don't any of you want to get out of the car? Addie, come on over here and help me with wheelie."

"Wait'll you see the Cuckoo Brothers and their crazy wheelie machine, Mangie!" Adam says.

Mother immediately clasps her hands in front of her bosom in the pose of delighted anticipation.

I get out of the car and go to open Pete's door.

"I see you've put on a little weight, Mary-Lou," she says, "especially around the hips."

Adam unfolds the chair expertly, pressing on the inside edges of the seat. He lugs the heavy gel-filled cushion over from the trunk and settles it in place. Next he squats to slip in the hinges to attach the leg rests to the chair, and swings them into position. Finally he stands up, leans over and locks the brakes against the wheels by pulling stoutly down on each of two rubber-covered levers. He double-checks the levers. Only nine years old, and he cannot afford to be careless.

Larry reaches in the car for Pete, scoops him up from the upholstery, and in one smooth motion, lowers him softly into the chair. Adam grips the handles, steps on the back chrome struts and from them climbs, first one foot, then the other, on top of the big black wheels, riding astride the wheelchair like an acrobat about to stand up on the back of a horse.

"Ta-daa!" Adam cries, letting go of the handles, straightening up and stretching his arms out wide. "It's the Cuckoo Brothers and their crazy wheelie machine!"

"The Cuckoo Brothers and their crazy, *possessed* wheelie machine!" Peter joins in, gripping the armrests, ready for action.

It starts softly; hardly a sound at all. More a sense of something having changed behind my back; complicated, emphatic, expectant, like the sound made by an orchestra readying its instruments, lifting fiddles to chins, reeds to lips, in response to the maestro's command.

Irregular, husky sounds, as intimate as the grunts of passion, startle the air. The hairs rise on my arms. Bewildered, I turn around.

Mother stands in the driveway, stricken, her fingertips pressed against her cheekbones, her eyes staring, her mouth open. "Oh, spare me this, dear God, it's more than I can bear," she murmurs over and over again, her shoulders heaving.

In a second I am at her, yanking her hands from her face, shaking her by the shoulders, holding her up against the side of the car as if I would frisk her of all feeling.

"You stop crying this instant, do you hear me?" I hiss each word separately, with venomous exactitude, straight into her face. "Don't you dare cry," I threaten as I lead her around the car, open the door and put her in.

"Don't you ever cry over my child again in front of him!" I say as I slam the door.

"Is that any way to talk to your mother?" she sniffles and shifts into reverse.

"What can I do to get back at him, Adam, what can I do?" Peter bends forward in his wheelchair, and using the lower part of his arm as a lever, the table's edge as the fulcrum, swings a forkful of steak at his mouth.

"What's the kid's name?" Adam asks.

"Tony."

"Tony who?"

"Tony Pinelli."

"Is Tony Pinelli an Italian name, Dad?" Adams asks.

"I think so. Why?"

"Then call him a wop," says Adam, setting his milk glass down with a clunk and wiping his mouth with the back of his hand.

"A *what?*" I exclaim.

"A wop," Adam repeats.

"Look, guys"—I set down my fork and knife for emphasis—"you don't call people names based on their nationality. It's cruel and stupid. I don't want you teaching such words to Peter, and I don't want you using them yourself."

"But I want to be cruel," says Peter. "I want to hurt his feelings."

"Well," says Larry, "you'll have to find some other way to get back at him."

"What did Tony Pinelli do to you?" I ask, fearing the worst. "Did he call you a bad name?"

"No."

"Well, then, what did he do?"

"He came up to me in the hall in between classes, locked the brakes on my wheelchair and left me stranded. I hate my wheelie." Pete begins to cry. "It's like a jail. I feel alone, as if the whole world is walking away from me."

"Oh, Petie," I sigh, reaching to rest my hand on his arm as if my touch could draw the hurt out of him like a poultice. "What an awful thing to do."

"Let Pete call him a wop, c'mon," Adam urges.

"Forget it," says Larry. "I think we should all put our heads together and find a good way to help Peter with his problem. Now," he says, warming to the task, "what is it we want to accomplish?"

"We want to make him stop," says Pete eagerly, the tears still damp on his cheeks.

"And we want revenge," Adam adds. "We want to make him suffer. Right, Pete?"

"Right!"

"Suppose you tell the principal," I suggest. "I'm sure he'd give Tony a punishment, or at least a warning. I know Dr. Christianson would appreciate your reporting the incident. You'd be doing it to help the other handicapped kids in the school too, not just yourself. After all, I bet other kids get teased unfairly too, don't they?"

Peter nods.

"Well, then, see? You'd be a hero." I've almost got myself convinced, but the stony silence that awaits my suggestion reminds me that kids who tell the principal are creeps.

"I want to *do* something," says Peter.

"I know," I answer. "I don't blame you. Let's think some more. Something besides bad names and hitting."

"Those are the only good things," says Adam advisedly.

"I wonder"—Larry tips back in his chair—"if Tony Pinelli has given a moment's thought to what a mean thing he's doing. What if you said something to him, Pete?"

Peter shakes his head.

"Hear me out, Pierre. I know it's asking a lot of you, maybe more than is fair from someone not quite ten, but suppose you explained to Tony that locking the brakes on your wheelchair is the same as if you went over to him and broke his legs."

"I couldn't do that," says Peter solemnly. "You were right. It's too much to expect from a child my age."

"I know what!" Adam exclaims, souping up excitement and hope in Pete's discouraged face. "What about a different version of Daddy's idea? Suppose you go up to Tony in school tomorrow and you say, 'Tony, I have something to tell you. Locking the brakes on my wheelchair is the same as if I broke both your legs. So if you ever lock my brakes again, my brother will find you and break both your legs.' How's that for an idea, buddy boy?"

"It's good," beams Peter.

"It's better than wop," Larry whispers in my ear.

"Happy Birthday to you, Happy Birthday to you!" We all start out on different notes, in spite of rehearsals in the master bathroom, where we designated ourselves the Crap Family singers, but by the second "to you" we seem to have agreed upon a key. That's when we crash into the brown tin humidifier that projects into the hallway, just outside the bathroom leading to Peter's room.

"Shit!" hisses Adam, who's riding on Larry's lap, naked except for the underpants he sleeps in now that puberty is percolating. Larry, who sleeps completely naked, is driving nude. I am riding on the back in my nightgown.

"It takes some getting used to," says Larry, backing away

from the wall in frantic little rabbit hops and lurches that culminate in a dervish of a 360-degree whirl.

"Keep singing," he admonishes, fumbling with the controls, but Adam and I are laughing too hard to sing.

"Shhh!" Larry turns on us sternly. "You'll wake him up!"

"Why don't we put it on manual, disengage the motors and just push it into his room," I whisper.

"That'll spoil all the fun!" Adam is exasperated. "Don't give up, Daddy."

Fortified by filial encouragement and confidence, Larry presses the joy stick and sends 250 pounds of stainless-steel wheelchair and lead batteries hurtling into the toilet.

"Do you really think a ten-year-old is going to be able to drive this," Larry asks, recovering from the indignity, "if I can't?"

On the kitchen wall, behind beveled glass, the long, trembling black arms of the pendulum clock are spread-eagled, one hand pinioned just above the three; the other flattened up against the ten. It is 2:50 P.M. Ten minutes of Peter. All the vectors of my day converge upon this moment.

I tell my life in time. I have to be up at 6:30 in order to get Peter ready in time for the school bus. If I haven't heard his voice, gruff with sleep, calling "Mom" over the intercom, I head for the kitchen to make coffee, even before I pee. On my way, I see that Larry has already occupied the bathroom. He sits on the toilet, pencil poised, the *New York Times* drawn and quartered on his lap.

"What's a four-letter word for a Ugandan exile?"

"Go fuck yourself."

If Peter has already called, I go directly to his room, lift the covers off his head, unwrap his arms from around Soft Gray, his lamb's-wool hippo, roll him over on his back if he is sleeping on his side, and kiss him good morning on his bellybutton. Then I hold the urinal while he pees, which reminds me that I haven't.

Then I exercise his limbs, lifting first one leg, folding and unfolding it, chanting to Petie all the while, "Open and close, open and close; that's the boy, help me—good, that's *good*—open and close, open and close." And then I put it down and pick up the other leg, and then one arm, and then the other arm, sensing with my muscles whether or not he is using his. Sometimes I can't even tell.

"Come on, Petie, *help!*"

"I *am!*"

We do that for about ten minutes. In order to keep on schedule, I've got to begin dressing him by 6:40. That takes another ten minutes, what with raveling out each sleeve and each trouser leg in my hands and threading each limb through, the way I used to dress my dolls.

Then I call Larry because I can't put Peter into the wheelchair. I'm strong enough to lift him from wheelchair to bed, but the other way around takes more control than I have. Peter weighs as much as I do.

"Laaaaa-ry! Laaaaa-ry!" I call over the distant sound of a toilet flushing. "Pete's ready to get into his chair." This morning our timing is elegant. I got him right between the first two of the three big *S*'s: shit, shave and shower.

" 'Morning, Potsie." Larry strolls in naked and smiling. "Ready to get into your chair?" He says it as if getting into the wheelchair were a joint effort, as if they depended upon each other.

I stand back while Larry bends over Peter, slides his left arm behind his back, insinuates his right hand between the backs of his knees and the bed.

"Ready?"

"Ready."

"One, two, three . . . up!" In one smooth motion, Larry picks him up and lowers him gently into the chair, finishing with a ritual kiss behind Peter's ear.

We've got to be in the bathroom by 6:50. The first thing I do is push up his cuffs and balance his arms on the edge of the sink. Then I turn on the water and wait until it flows warm against the inside of my wrist.

"Are you sure it's not too hot?" Peter always asks. I burned him once.

I soap my hands, turning the bar over and over in my palms until they are lavish with lather. Then I take Peter's limp little hands and move them about in mine as if they were slivers of soap. I hold them under the faucet to rinse, leaving them there while I reach for the towel. Peter loves the feel of the water. Then I pat them dry on a towel, pull down the cuffs, put his elbows on his armrests and his hands in his lap.

Time to wash his face. I put a towel around Pete's shoulders and one on his lap to keep his clothes from getting wet because he can't lean forward over the sink. I carry soapy water to his face on a washcloth in my palm. The clock in the kitchen begins to bong seven as I am patting his face dry.

As the clock chimes its last, Adam tries to open the bathroom door from the hallway, but it bangs into the back wheels of Peter's chair.

"Sorry!" he acknowledges. "I'll come through the other way."

Adam enters the bathroom through Peter's room, stands at the toilet and pees, reminding me that I still haven't. In the distance I hear the familiar metallic clunk followed by the rush and syncopated beat of the shower set on "massage."

"So much for shit and shave," I mutter.

"Great! I'll go take a shower with Daddy!" Adam yells, flushing the toilet with his foot and leaping over the back wheels of Pete's chair and out the door. "See ya!"

It's already after seven and I still haven't brushed his teeth. "Open up!" I always start in the back on the bottom around the lower molars, and brush first around the outsides and then around the insides. Then I move to the upper jaw. Up, inside, in the back is the hardest place to get at in somebody else's mouth. "Open wider!"

"Ooooow!" Peter cries out testily from his wide-open mouth. "Hat hurts!"

"Oh, come on, now, that didn't hurt," I conclude, taking the brush from his mouth and running it under the water. "Go hocktooey." Peter loves to spit. He gives it his all. I see a tiny strand of pink in the fine white foam. I did hurt him.

By the time Pete's at his place and I lift his hands onto the table, it's 7:05. We'll have to hurry through breakfast. I'll have to help him eat.

By 7:20 he's got to be done eating because he wants to pee again, even though he just had a big pee an hour ago, because he hopes that if he can get rid of every drop at home, maybe he won't have to pee in school. But of course he will. He knows that. But, still . . .

Between 7:20 and 7:30, when the bus comes, is time for putting on his hat and coat and especially the knitted gloves that keep his hands warm while he drives his chair. Even though I stretch them wide open at the wrist and lower them carefully, and even though Peter cooperates by holding his hand as up as he can and by spreading his fingers wide, just so, we sometimes end up with an uninhabited glove finger, as flat and limp as a milked-out teat.

At 7:30 Larry emerges from the bedroom a lawyer, the way Clark Kent steps out of a phone booth, just in time to roll Peter over the threshold onto the ramp, while I hold the storm door open.

"So long Fudgickle-Pudgickle, have a terrific day! I'll see you at dinner!" Larry calls and waves as the bus backs out of the driveway. Then he heads for his car.

"Don't you want some coffee?" I call from the door.

"I've got to run," Larry answers over the roof of his car. "I'm on trial."

Seven thirty-five is when I pee.

Right after that is when I notice that Adam has left without eating any breakfast.

For the next hour I move like a water bug over the surface

of my life, darting, turning, crossing my own path, addicted to my own speed, my own moving target. When I leave the house for *Fairpress* at 8:45 the beds are made, the breakfast dishes are done, dinner is a frosted rock on the counter, my heart is pounding, and there is sweat on my upper lip.

Nine o'clock is when I get to *Fairpress,* lift the cover off my typewriter as if it were a magic act, insert a piece of yellow copy paper in the roller and begin to write my humor column.

"A funny thing happened on the way to the office . . ." I sometimes write, just to warm up my fingers while I'm waiting for an idea, the way other people type "the quick brown fox . . ."

The only time all day that I don't know what time it is, is when the keys begin to touch themselves—or am I really playing them, like some literary E. Power Biggs at the mighty Royal Standard—in any case, it's happening, this intentional spontaneity, this scientific magic. I soar, I plunge, I'm lost, I'm found, I'm writing!

Two-thirty is when I cover my typewriter like a canary for the night and burn rubber down the Post Road, racing Peter home, swearing behind the flashing backs of yellow school buses. Home, where dinner lies on the counter in a pool of blood, and the clock in the kitchen says two-fifty. I made it.

Ready or not, here he comes. Like clockwork.

What'll I do? What'll I do? Whadil I do? Whadilido? Whadil? I panic at the thought of so much time between now and when Larry and Adam come home for dinner, filling the house with pace and a sense of the world. So much time to be in charge of, to fill, to spend, to be crushed by.

Leaning against the sidelights in the front hall, as if stage-struck, anticipating and dreading the sound of the bus as it labors up Sturges Commons, I pray that Peter is in a good mood.

Here he comes! The school bus, gaudy as a marigold, turns into the oak-lined driveway, its tires against the gravel making the sound of crushed bones. The leaves and branches slap and clatter against the roof of the bus as it cuts its own canopy. I watch as the driver climbs out of his seat, crosses in front of the van and activates the sliding side door with a quick downward jerk.

I can hardly see Peter behind the cagelike metal grating of the folding ramp, which fills the doorway opening, but I know he is in there, facing backwards like a prisoner. The large back wheels of his chair press against the back of the driver's seat and are sunk into two-inch-deep metal grooves in the floor, held in place, against quick stops and starts, with locking pins.

How will he be? I try to see him, to study him, to prepare for him, before he sees me. I peer through the sidelights, my breath ebbing and flowing, silently etching vaporous waves on the cold glass pane. Like a diver, snatching one last gulp of air before descending, my heart indulges in one more swell of sorrow for this child, teacher-dressed, who waits patiently to be undone.

The driver unfolds the ramp, which clatters and falls open with an alarming crash and then settles its metal lip against the asphalt. The bus driver climbs the corrugated ramp in his rubber-soled boots, which hardly ever slip, and bends down on his knees on the floor of the van in front of Peter. No words are spoken as he reaches under the seat of the wheelchair and fumbles to unslip the pins that attach the backs of the big wheels to the floor. Then he stands up, reaches to one side, pulls the lever to disengage the drive belts, grabs hold of the rubber-handled wheelchair grips, hauls Peter out of the wheel wells and drags the chair backwards, tugging right and left, until the back wheels are lined up with the top of the ramp. After a brief pause to catch his breath, he pulls backwards on the handles and, at the same time, leans his weight forward against the chair's downward rolling momentum, like some reverse Sisyphus whose rock has turned against him.

At the bottom of the ramp he turns the chair to face the house, steps back, turns and reaches down to fold the ramp, first once upon itself and then, with one final upward heave, upright, where it locks in place. A snap of his wrist, and the door slides closed with a whoosh and a satisfying clench.

"Engage me and turn my wheelchair on," I hear Pete say. That is enough for me to know he's in a bad mood. He usually says, "I'm lovely, I'm disengaged, I use Pond's." It's one of my jokes he's made his own. The driver turns, pulls back on the lever, flicks the toggle switch to "on" and says, "Goodbye, Pete. See you tomorrow."

Pete is already having trouble turning on his wheelchair. I begin to invent a device, like an elevator call button, that operates at a mere touch—I, who do not understand why electricity doesn't flow out of an abruptly unplugged cord like water from a hose—and I decide to find a good electrician.

Still not time to step out from the wings. I watch through the pane as Peter steers around the edge of the garden that separates the front of the house from the turnaround. I see him gun the joy stick forward and lower his head like a linebacker as he turns right and approaches the bottom of the concrete ramp, which runs along the front of the house, inclining ten degrees each linear foot, past the bay window, and levels out to form a landing at the front door.

I move away from the sidelights, open the door and come to life. "Sorry," I say, shaking my head back and forth and looking gruff, "we are not expecting any special deliveries. Perhaps you belong to the house next door. What's your name, kid?"

"I'm not in the mood to fool around," Peter announces sternly, shooting right through the front door, zooming past my toes as I stand crucified in the doorway, one arm flattened against the storm door, holding it out, the other against the front door, holding it in.

Peter bee-lines through the entrance hall, through the kitchen, almost grazing the lower cabinets with a leg rest as he veers deftly right, then left, to position himself, and drives straight under his place at the kitchen table and throws the joy stick into reverse too late, coming to a stop only after his stomach, on impact, nudges the table, which makes a growling noise as it grates a few inches across the floor.

"Sorry," says Pete. "I'm in a bad mood."

"Speaking of pissed, would you like to?" One more joke, just one more, to see if it will make a difference.

"Okay," he says, pulling back on the joy stick to back out from under the table, "but first take off my clothes. Hurry up. I gotta go bad." He swings the side of his foot impatiently against the bar of the leg rest, making a tapping sound. I notice that his sneaker is coming off at the heel. Peter's Achilles tendons are becoming more and more foreshortened, pulling his heels upward, pointing his toes to the floor. I try on the word "deformed." Someone must make shoes for deformed feet. I make a mental note to look into that.

"You shouldn't hold it in so long, Pierre. Why don't you ask your teacher to piss you before you leave school each day?" I ask, knowing the answer, as I hasten to unzip his baseball jacket and lift first one arm aloft by the knit cuff and then the other, letting gravity take over, slipping his arm limply through, leaving an empty sleeve. He leans forward, and I snatch the jacket out from behind him and head down the hall toward the bathroom like a stunt pilot, tipping my wings. Pausing briefly to hang the jacket up on its hook outside his room with one hand, I level off as I glide through his room and out into the bathroom, where I tip my wing to pluck the urinal from the back of the toilet with the other before coming back down the hall for a landing at my point of departure.

I work my thumb and first two fingers under the elastic waistband of his pants and pull outward and down, making enough space in his crotch to slip the urinal under his penis.

"Ow!" he yowls sharply. "Can't you be more careful?"

"I'm sorry," I wince, anguished for this child, angry with this brat, who will not be cheered.

"I'm sorry," he says. "It's just that everybody's always doing that. It hurts terribly. You don't have a dickie. You don't know."

"You're right. But I can imagine."

"Here it comes," he sighs, rolling his head back. Always a shy stranger to this intimate moment, I watch his eyebrows arch, his nostrils dilate, his eyelids reach and stretch closed.

"Ecstasy," he murmurs, "sheer ecstasy." The odor of his urine wafts into my nostrils. I accept it with the same mixture of relish and disgust as I do my own.

"Okay," I say, moving right along, when the piss is flushed, the Lysol spray is aimed down the neck of the urinal, and Peter is tucked into his place at the kitchen table. "What do you want for snack today?"

I open up the pantry doors and look inside. "We've got apricots, raisins, half-dill pickles"—his favorites. "Remember, you're on a diet, Fudgickle-Pudgickle." There is also a box of D-Zerta low-cal gelatin dessert. I haven't made it yet. The saccharin cancer warning displayed prominently on the side panel by government decree puts me off every time. This time, what the hell, I reach for the box. Peter's been granted a special dispensation. Muscular dystrophy will get him before cancer can.

The diet was Dr. Braverman's idea. "He's getting too fat, Mary-Lou. We can't let him get fat."

"Why not, Hal? Why the hell not?"

"Because it's unhealthy."

"For Chrissakes, Hal. *Unhealthy?*"

"Peter's respiration already tests three-quarters of normal. That means the muscles of his lungs and diaphragm are being affected. That apron of fat on his belly is actually exerting pressure upward on his diaphragm, inhibiting breathing. Can you still lift him?"

"Just barely," I confessed.

"That's another good reason for him to take off twenty pounds."

"Twenty pounds?" My voice rose. "Is he that much overweight?" I guess he is. I never see him that way, the way everyone else must see him. Twenty pounds. He must be fat. He may even be grotesque. "I hate to put him on a diet. He loves to eat. It's one of his favorite things to do, besides drawing. He has so little left!"

"I'm sorry, Mary-Lou."

"How about apricots? He loves apricots." Already I was bargaining.

"They're okay. You could try diet gelatin. He might like that."

"But no Oreos?"

"No Oreos."

"I'll make you some Jell-O for dinner tonight," I propose, turning away from the pantry toward Peter, shaking the box in the air.

"Don't put any fruit in it."

"Why not?"

"It feels like I'm eating the end of my nose."

"Okay, no fruit. Now, what do you want for snack?"

"Are the apricots the plump or the wrinkled kind?"

"The plump kind." I know that is the wrong answer. "I couldn't find any wrinkled ones. I went to three different stores. Only plump ones."

"I hate the plump ones. How about an Oreo?" he leers.

"How about a punch in the snoot?"

"How about two Oreos?"

"How about a bribe? You quit being in a bad mood and I'll give you an Oreo. Dr. Spock says if you can get the desired results by bribing a kid, you should feel free."

"Who's Dr. Spock?"

"He's a famous pediatrician who writes books for parents about how to raise their kids."

"It also says you should give a kid two Oreos after school."

"Where does it say that?" I ask.

"In *The Book of Kids,*" Pete answers neatly.

"What else does it say in *The Book of Kids*?" I ask.

"Lots. It talks about bedtimes, and then there's a whole

chapter about cottage cheese," says Peter, who hates it.

"Where do you keep this book? May I see it?"

"It's been mis-be-placed. I don't know where it is."

"So do we have a deal? Are you bribed?" I set a glass of skim milk in front of him and stick in a straw. I place the open bag of Oreos near his hand, remove one and hold the cookie behind my back to make it more exciting. "Only one."

"Okay." Peter opens up his mouth and thrusts out his tongue. His tongue is the strongest muscle. He likes to use it. "Hut hit hin, hlease."

"Here hit his," I tease, laying it on.

He retracts his tongue swiftly, cashing the cookie in as if it were a penny on the red tin tongue of a clown on an antique toy bank. I watch his jaws crunch down and then turn my back and walk toward the sink. Even though my back is turned, I know that right now his fingers are creeping, dragging his palm behind them across the pine table toward the open bag. The sound of crinkling cellophane confirms that Pete is snitching. I wait until he has had time to lean back in his chair, giving him enough leverage to slide the cookie toward him. By now it must be at the table's edge. He will lean his forearms on the table and lower his head until he can grab the cookie with his mouth. Then, cookie clenched between his teeth, he will press against the table with his arms and struggle to right himself in his chair. He may have to try twice. I give him extra time.

I whirl around to meet his bad-boy grin. Brown crumbs cling to his lips. "You rascal! You thief! You common criminal, lower than the low, sneakier than the sneakiest, badder than the bad!" Like a parody of an old lady chasing after a purse snatcher, I run across the kitchen floor, grab the bag of cookies from the table, stuff it in the pantry and slam the bifold doors while Peter wiggles and giggles in his wheelchair.

I pull out my chair and sit down next to him at the table. The after-school ceremonies have ended on a high note; now we're on our own. I glance at the clock. Only three. Well, moving right along . . .

"What do you feel like doing today?" I ask, as if being ten years old and having no friends to play with except me, and no place to be except home, and no body to play with, except just a head and hands, were a prospect rich with possibilities.

"How about let's take a walk?" I've almost gotten over seeing the irony in that. Once we joked about taking a "roll," but it didn't stick. We take walks.

"I don't feel like taking a walk today. I'm not in the mood."

"Well, then, maybe you're tired. How about let's play a board game?"

"I hate board games. They make me bored."

Moving right along . . . "Maybe you're in the mood to watch a little TV"—I hope, I hope, I hope.

"Bor-ing," he sing-songs, replicating perfectly the interval and intonation of the Avon lady's door chimes. "Besides," he adds, "there's nothing on at this time except The Pain and Strife of Family Life." That's Peter's generic term for soap operas.

"Do you want to listen to records in your room?"

"No."

"Well, then," I hear myself say and can tell right away that I am getting annoyed, annoyed that this child, of all children, will not like anything passive, will not give up, "do you feel like reading?"

"No."

"That leaves drawing." The old stand-by.

"Okay," he says with a sigh. "Will you draw too?"

"Sure I will." I try to generate a little enthusiasm to offset the gravity pull of my depression and his, which makes me yearn to settle into the cushy velvet sofa in the living room, pull my knees up under my chin and flip through the pages of *Time* magazine, scrounging and picking like a chimp for vicarious morsels of life in the People section. "I'll get us some paper and pencils," I say, getting up from my chair and going over to the kitchen desk. I glance up at the bulletin board and notice that I've forgotten to subscribe to series tickets at the Long Wharf Theater. Chalk up another inadvertent surrender.

"Don't forget my ruler," says Pete.

I open the desk drawer and take a stack of paper; his six-inch ruler (a twelve-inch is too hard for him to handle); two pencils, a No. 1 for him and a No. 2 for me. Now Peter can make only faint gray lines with a No. 2. As I insert his pencil into the electric sharpener and wait until the grating noise diminishes into a smooth hum, I wonder if they make anything softer than a No. 1. I'll have to find out. It's easier for him if the pencil is very sharp. The ruler, I suppose, is to fence in a world of his own creation, a world of power and motion, under his sole control. He always draws cars.

"What are you going to draw?"

"A car."

"What kind of a car?"

"A fast one, a Maserati. What are you going to draw?"

"I think I'll draw you drawing a Maserati. Is that all right with you?"

Peter doesn't answer. He is already at work. He is revving up: *"Vvvvvvvroooom, vvvroom."*

His right hand holds the pencil delicately, like a chopstick held in place more by balance than strength. It moves in small, slow increments against the ruler's edge, guided, it seems, by small, swift thrusts from the tip of his tongue, which protrudes intently near one corner of his mouth.

The fingers of his left hand rest on the ruler. The tips are nearly translucent, as if this were where the strength flows out of him, subcutaneously. The nails are innocent, fetal. The fingers are thin, white, effete; almost bony. The fat of boyhood is gone.

I begin to sketch them in faintly as they lie, splayed out, holding the ruler down. Dimples indent where knuckles should protrude. His hands are turning inside out, his fingers are curving backwards, like petals about to fall from a flower. I examine his wrists and arms; they are girlishly thin and juvenile, almost vestigial. They are too young and shapeless for his barrel-chested torso and large head. His body is not growing up.

Peter is dying from the outside in, diminishing, infantalizing from the tips of his fingers and the ends of his toes. Everywhere, except his head.

"Muscular. I assume that part is clear enough," I hear Dr. Braverman say. "Self-explanatory, actually. Now dystrophy. Dystrophy refers to the atrophying of the muscles in a distended position." All over. From the tips of his fingers. Everywhere. Except the head.

I draw from his head toward his hands. His auburn hair has darkened, thickened and curled, losing its childish fineness to the beginnings of adolescence. His nose, once fleshy and pert, is taking on the seriousness of a bony structure building beneath, although freckles still look at home, especially on the cheeks, round though not so pink. I notice a bit of adult shadow beneath each lowered eye and smudge the pencil lines with the edge of my thumb.

Peter is changing, growing up and dying down, into a new kind of beauty—mutant, contradictory, promising and ominous. I finish the drawing at his fingertips, touching each one with the tip of the eraser.

"Oh God"—I compose a prayer over Peter's image—"it's me again. Look, maybe I've been asking for too much. How about something more modest. It's true. I am not a believer. I shouldn't expect you to look kindly upon me. I know you've got a lot of faithful adherents who, if you're anything like people, you'd much rather be nice to than me. But on the other hand, I can't help but think that if you really are God, you're better than people. That's the whole point, isn't it? You shouldn't have grudges against people like me. So, if you won't save his life, would you please consider saving his fingers? Please? He loves to draw. See? He's drawing a car right now. No big deal. Will you please, God, just make his fingers last as long as he does?"

"I'm finished." Peter lets the pencil roll out of his hand and flicks the ruler away with his fingertips. "Do you like it?"

"I love it!"

"It's aerodynamically sound"—Pete reads a lot of automotive magazines—"and it has many optional features. See the inflatable air bag? Here's the telescoping steering wheel which collapses on impact. They're both advanced safety features."

Safety. Peter worries about safety.

"Does it have any cam shafts?" I ask, trying to get into the swing.

"Sure. Lots of them. And it has retrorockets and wire wheels and a roll bar and it goes five thousand miles per hour and forty million revolutions per minute. It's the fastest car in the world. I'm going to have one if I grow up."

My eyes widen to hold their light and my mouth strains to keep its smile while the blood drains from my face. "Maybe by the time you grow up they'll have even faster cars," I reply brazenly over the gnawing in my chest, and I wonder if he knows—if somewhere, in the back of his mind or the tips of his fingers, he knows that time is running out.

"Maybe. Turn on my wheelchair, please. I want to listen to records in my room. Don't take the pencil," he cautions as I move to put away the drawing materials. "I like to bang it against my bureau in time to the music. I'm a rock star."

"Is my hair neat or messy?" Peter asks as I put his favorite Beatles record on the phonograph in his room.

"Neat."

"Good, because my favorite thing to pretend is that I'm playing for an audience of three hundred thousand and I want my hair to be neat, you know, to protect my image." He shoots me one of those I-know-I'm-being-a-little-silly-for-my-age looks but-it's-so-much-fun-let's-just-let-ourselves-be-silly-even-though-we-know-better—okay?

"Ladies and gentlemen, now onstage at Madison Square Garden, direct to you from Liverpool, Peter Weisman and the Beatles!" I announce as the record drops onto the turntable with a clunk, and the arm, as if enchanted, hovers, then alights on the record's edge. I watch to make sure that the needle has slipped into the groove before I withdraw from his room backwards, bent at the waist like an impresario, one arm extended in a flourishing "Ta-daa!" in his direction. He waits at the bureau's edge for the music to start, his pencil poised and a faraway look in his eyes.

I sit back down at the kitchen table and lay my head on my arms. Two nights of insomnia. I am exhausted.

I'd better face it. I'm trying to do too much. I've got to quit my job at *Fairpress*.

The kitchen clock whirrs and strikes four.

"It's been a hard day's night," the Beatles are singing. Peter is tapping.

"I bet he could play the drums," I think to myself, staring over the top of my arm, and make a note to look into it.

"You've got to take care of yourself," I hear Sara's voice in my mind.

I make a note to look into that, too.

Leaning against the door frame in the hotel lobby, I wonder if they can tell that I'm an impostor, a housewife among working women, a weakling among Amazons, a nearly totaled woman in a roomful of feminists.

I observe the women as they go, in and out of the conference room, talking about whether a journalist who calls herself a feminist ought to write for the women's page of a newspaper, even if the page is now called the Style page; sexual harassment at the water cooler; and who is and is not here at the annual, jointly sponsored Liebling MORE/NOW Writer's Conference.

I am a dead giveaway, dressed as I am in my pitiful, shamefully skewed idea of what the up-to-date New York feminist-journalist is wearing: a white silk blouse with a large, soft pussycat bow at the throat, to soften the otherwise too severe lines of my executive suit.

I hang back against the entrance to the conference room, examining each woman's face for telltale signs of fulfilled potential, listening to their voices for that reassuring timbre, that cadence of easy self-confidence that denotes a genuine feminist—and it takes everything I've got not to bolt from the lobby, tear down Forty-third Street in my low-heeled, high-minded executive pumps, which absolutely no one is wearing, and grab the next train back to Westport.

I should have known. I can never be one of them. I am one of those unlucky born-too-early women aged forty or more over whose bodies the feminists will march on their triumphant way to liberation, whose fate it is to long for, but never get to, the Promised Land.

Like the Biblical scapegoat bearing the sins of an entire people, banished forever into the wilderness, it is my lot to carry the sins of my sexist sisters—the faked orgasms, the unchanged flat tires, the teased cocks—into exile. There I will live out my days, cursed by my own half-raised consciousness; doomed to act like a cunt, and to know better. And in that unfortunate order.

Even Nora Ephron can't help me. I heard her speak earlier this morning on the subject of how to begin a career in freelancing for magazines. She said what I was afraid she would say.

"In order to get started in freelance writing for magazines, you must first have a freelance article published in a magazine." Ms. Ephron wrinkles her cute nose, shrugs her slim shoulders and smiles wryly, letting the audience know that the irony is intentional.

The situation is pretty discouraging, she quite agrees, although she doesn't look particularly discouraged. Why should she? She is the darling of her sorority, the well-scrubbed feminist next-door type, the Debbie Reynolds of the women's movement, and she's about to marry her Eddie Fisher update, Carl Bernstein—small, dark, and investigative.

"Does it help to have an agent?"

The answer is no. Besides, you can't get an agent until you've at least had something published. And you can't get something published until you've gotten something published.

In sum, you can't get there from here.

I might as well give up and go home.

The speaker mounted over the doorway to the conference room crackles, coughs and emits an electronic high note, as piercingly neural as the sound of chalk on the blackboard, uniting all the women, for one moment, in one vast, aggregate shudder. "Will you please take your seats? The open mike portion of this morning's program is about to begin. Sorry about the noise," she adds, soothing acres of goose flesh.

I stand, paralyzed as usual, like a child playing musical chairs and needing to win too much. I watch the women move in from the lobby and scramble for the remaining vacant seats. I hang back and wait until there is only one seat left, way in the back, and no one but me left standing.

What the hell, I'll stay, even though I know it's not really my game. What the hell, I'll just hang in and watch them bat their viable options around.

I know how Peter must feel when he is invited to join a baseball game by Adam and his well-meaning friends who are determined that he shall not be an outcast—that, somehow, he shall play with them. Peter always ends up keeping score.

Looking more like a madam than a chairwoman, a big blowsy blonde, wearing red tights and spike heels, wraps her hand tentatively around the base of the microphone, eyes it warily and licks her lips, as if she were considering fellatio.

"Is the mike on?" she asks, pauses and then smiles with relief. The microphone is going to behave itself. "We'll conduct this hour-long part of the program very informally. Those of you who wish to speak, form a line at the mike; and please limit the length of your remarks so that everyone who wishes will have a turn. This is your opportunity to make announcements or ask questions."

A slim, bright-eyed brunette heads up the line. She holds a clipboard to her chest and leans into the microphone like an Andrews sister. "All women journalists who think they have been discriminated against by their employers and who would like to consider forming a legal action group, please meet with me after the open mike at one P.M., in suite 246." She lowers her clipboard into writing position. "May I see a show of hands of those women who think they might be interested in attending?" She appraises the raised hands, conducting the silent count with her pencil. "Thank you very much. Remember, that's one o'clock, suite 246. Next?" She walks away from the mike.

If I had an announcement, I wonder, what would it be?

"All women journalists who have children who are dying, who have had to quit the jobs they love, and who may not survive the deaths of their children unless they can hang on to some life of their own, something that cannot die, will all such women please meet with me at two P.M. in suite 535 for a quick game of Russian roulette? May I see a show of hands?"

And if I had a question, I wonder, what would it be?

"Sisters, can you help me?"

A smiling, robust woman who might have hiked off the pages of an L. L. Bean catalog, the kind you're almost positive must have some very unlikely profession—an embalmer, perhaps—on *What's My Line?*, takes her turn at the mike.

"My name is Shirley Smith Anderson. I live in Princeton, New Jersey. I produce a newspaper column called 'One Woman's Voice,' which is syndicated by the *New York Times* and appears weekly in about eighty newspapers nationwide. Our regular columnists include Abigail McCarthy, Nikki

Giovanni and Clare Boothe Luce, among others. The columns are rotated weekly, so that each woman writes about one column per month, for which I pay the paltry sum of one hundred and fifty dollars. I'm sorry I can't afford to pay more. I am hopeful that as soon as we sell to a few more papers, I'll be in a position to offer two hundred dollars.

"I am looking for a woman who can write a humor column once a month. I don't mean the usual domestic humor, either, the 'a funny thing happened to me on the way to the dryer, or at the Little League game,' although I agree that Erma Bombeck is often funny. I'm looking for a female humorist with a broader range. She need not consider herself a feminist. We're not even sure we're a feminist syndication, but we're sure that we're humanists. I always calm the fears of editors, still frightened of women with opinions, by telling them that we are not the flying syndicated wedge of the women's movement, even though we really are when feminists speak out in the column.

"There are very few good women humorists. I can count them on the fingers of one hand. Is there a woman here who thinks she can fill the bill? If so, I'd like to hear from her." Shirley Smith Anderson backs away from the microphone and threatens to disappear into the throng.

"I can!" I yell, standing up and waving. "I can!"

"Come on out!" I yell at the bathroom door and wiggle the knob. It's locked. The son of a bitch has locked himself in with the *Times* crossword puzzle. It's Sunday. Nine A.M. I've had it.

"I'll be out in a few minutes" comes the irritated reply.

"You're doing the crossword puzzle, aren't you? You know if you stay in there long enough, I will have to exercise Peter, dress Peter, wash Peter and cajole Peter into a good mood. I do it every goddamn day of the week. At least you could get Peter up on Sundays."

"Goddamn it, Mary-Lou, can't I even go to the bathroom in peace?"

"Peace he wants!" My tone changes from fishwife to Judy Holliday. "You're hiding. That's what you're doing, you coward. Let me in or I'll kick the door down!"

Through the door I hear him slap the paper down on the floor. "Do I have to justify my every move to you? What right have you to track me down in the bathroom?"

"How come you always stay in there just long enough to finish the crossword puzzle every Sunday? Go ahead, answer that one, counselor."

"I refuse to participate in this argument," says Larry. "Will you please get away from the door? I'll help you out with Peter as soon as I'm finished."

"Don't bother. As usual, I'm it. I've already dressed and exercised him. All-y, all-y in free. The coast is clear. You can come out now."

"You can be really vicious, Mary-Lou, you know that?"

"I didn't use to be vicious. I'm vicious from waking up twice each night while you snore like a pig next to me. I'm vicious from insomnia. Boy, can that make you vicious! You wouldn't know. I'm vicious because we made a deal before I took the job at *Fairpress*. You said you'd help me take care of Pete during the night and in the mornings, and in two whole years you've only done it six times."

"But who's keeping score."

"I gave up *Fairpress* and I'm not giving up the column. I need it."

"Look, I've told you a thousand times. Just wake me up. I don't hear Peter calling. It's not my fault. I just don't hear him. Give me a nudge, wake me up, and I'll be happy to turn him."

"Don't you understand? I don't want to be responsible. I don't want to have to wake you up. Besides, once I'm up, I'm up. I might as well do it myself. I want you to wake yourself up."

"I can't control that, for God's sake. I sleep soundly."

"You sleep soundly because you know I don't. You depend on it. If I weren't here one night, you'd wake up."

"Try me."

"That's not a bad idea."

"I do my fair share around here. You seem to forget I work for a living."

"Don't throw that old one up at me again. I'm sick of it. I'm sick of it, and I'm sick of your goddamn crossword puzzles, and I'm sick of you!" Now I am banging on the bathroom door with my fists. "I'm piling up hates on you, Larry. I'm not going to stay married to someone I hate. If I'm really as alone as I feel, then so be it. I'd rather know that now, and do something about it now. If you don't care enough about me, if all you care about is saving your own ass, then you can get the hell out of here!" I aim those last words, one by one, like darts, at the door.

The lock snaps. Larry opens the door. He stands there in his blue terrycloth robe, his arms hanging limply at his sides. "You're serious, aren't you?" He seems really surprised.

"Yes I am. Dead serious."

"I didn't realize you felt so strongly about this."

"Well, now you do. All I feel these days is strongly. I'm an emotional minefield. I'm sick of having all the feelings around here. I'm the heavy in this family, and I resent it. It's too great a burden, caring for him and resenting you. I'd rather just care for him. That would be a relief. Don't you understand what's happening? It's not enough for you to be a typical father and wage earner. Peter's not a typical kid. We're not a typical family. I'm not a typical mother. You can't go on behaving as if nothing is happening. And the funny thing is that you're missing something. Awful as it is at times, you're missing really knowing Peter. I know you love him, but I also know you're scared to get in too close, scared it'll hurt too much later on. I'm not going to let you get away with it. Maybe it's good for you, although I doubt it, but it sure as hell isn't good for me, and it isn't good for Peter. I want you to be in this as deeply as I am. So make up your mind. What'll it be? Are you in or out?"

Larry stands on the marble threshold between the bath-room and the hall, one hand resting on the doorknob, the other rubbing his weekend beard. "Is that what I've been doing?" he says after a while.

"That's what I think you've been doing. That's what I've been trying to tell you. That's what all our fights are about. I can't be any other way than the way that I am. I know I'm demanding. I know I make it hard for myself, but I can't do anything less for him than I can imagine. I just *can't*.

"I need to share this with you, Larry—not just the work—but the peril of loving him. It's terrifying to exchange so much love with someone who is going to die. It's a scary love, an archetypal love. Sometimes I feel so powerful, so heady, as if I were dancing on a ledge, leaping, nearly levitating, with the grace that his love gives me. And then, sometimes I wonder what the price is that I'll have to pay for having such a love, for stealing thunder from the gods. Of course I know. The price of having him is losing him."

"C'mere." Larry holds his arms out to me. I move toward him slowly and rest my cheek against the rough lapel of his robe. "I'm sorry," he says. "I didn't realize how much you were suffering. I didn't want to. We'll take turns getting up with Pete during the night. I'll take tonight. I'll do my best to hear him. I'll sleep on the side of the bed nearer to the in-tercom. I can't guarantee I'll hear him, but I'll try. And we'll take turns getting him dressed and ready for school in the mornings."

"Thank God," I whisper into the V of silky hairs on his chest. "At last! You are a very stubborn man, Larry Weis-man."

"You are getting to be quite a tough broad, Mary-Lou Weisman," he says, kissing my cheek. "You're right, you know. I *am* scared to get too close to Pete. I'm really not sure I can take it. You may, in spite of all your tears and emo-tional flamboyance, be the stronger one. I may just be the more stubborn."

I can tell by the way he is moving through the crowd in the lobby that Larry is pissed. He elbows, he bumps, he plunges, he butts, using his head and body like a broken field runner as he makes his way toward us, leaving a wake of unsettled theatergoers. A clutch of Helen Hokinson ladies stagger, regain their balance, and then draw themselves up to their full heights and look indignant daggers over their shoulders at his receding back. A Broadway party of four, catching a mere glance at the gathering storm voluntarily split asunder, then regroup to resume conversation with a shrug of their shoulders and the flick of a cigarette.

As he reaches us, the theater bell chimes.

"Sorry I'm late. The fucking parking lot attendant wouldn't let me park the van in his lot, even after I explained to him that it doesn't fit into any of the parking garages."

"Why wouldn't he take it?"

"Because it takes up more space than an average car for the same amount of money, that's why."

"Did you explain to him that the van was for a handicapped child? Maybe he would have been more sympathetic."

"Fuck him. I don't want his fucking sympathy."

"So where's the van?"

"I parked it in front of the entrance to his parking lot. And locked it!" His eyes flash triumph.

"For Chrissakes, Larry, the guy's just going to have you towed away, and it's going to be a big expensive pain in the ass. Just so you can get your rocks off."

"Of course I didn't *leave* the van there," Larry hastens to add, as if he had not intended to make that impression. "The attendant ran after me and told me I could park in the lot, after all. You've got to treat those sons of bitches like sons of bitches. That's all they understand. They're not interested in our personal plight. The world, in case you haven't noticed, is not a lovely place, and it sure as hell isn't our oyster."

"You could have tried. I hate all this anger—yours and mine. Anyhow, it's over. Let's find our seats before the lights go out."

"You asked for three orchestra seats next to the wheelchair space, didn't you?" the lady in the black dress with the white dickey inquires impatiently as she examines our stubs.

"Yes," I say, feeling the glossy *Playbills* grow sticky beneath my fingers. I test the tackiness with the ball of my thumb. "But no one bothered to mention that the handicapped seating was behind a three-foot-wide marble pillar and under the sound system. It's just not fair." I turn to Larry.

"We're not parking this child behind that pillar," says Larry. "He is going to see this show and hear this show just like everyone else in the theater."

"I'd better get the manager," she says.

"Good idea," says Larry, warming up. "I'll be happy to see him."

"Goody," says Adam. "We're going to have another fight."

Peter says nothing, and I wonder. Is he the hero, the soon-to-be-triumphant *cause célèbre* of this unfolding drama, or its pawn, its poster child of lost causes? I am afraid of what the world can do to him. Pete's face remains impassive. I cannot read it.

"It's against the fire laws to put him anywhere else," the manager explains, a thin veneer of the customer-relations courtesy course for theater managers holding his voice down.

I wonder how you get to be a theater manager. Do you start by wanting to be one or is it thrust upon you? Maybe you start as a movie usher, flashlight held high and trained downward, a matinée Diogenes looking for two together, not too close, while the Rockettes kick open the Warner-Pathé Newsreel, and I, holding my popcorn carefully against my chest, sashay in; excuse me, excuse me, excuse me, excuse me.

No, that's not it; ushers do not grow up to be theater managers. Movie ushers go on to better things, as soon as their acne clears up.

This one descended to the job, fell from something loftier, the near fulfillment of a lifelong dream, his own retail card shop or a Carvel franchise. An illusionless man. A dangerous man.

I notice that he has disregarded the label on his rumpled polyester plaid trousers and thrown them in the laundromat dryer on "High." The crease is nearly melted out. His jacket is from another suit. His fingers are white and stubby. He wears a high school ring with a dull red stone. He has an anonymous face. I have to keep looking at it to remember it.

"That's why we have special seating for the handicapped," he explains. "The law requires it."

"I'll say it's special," Adam mocks. "It's the worse seat in the house."

"Shhh," I warn. "Let Daddy handle this."

"Does the law," I say, turning toward the manager, "specify that people who must remain in their wheelchairs be guaranteed the worst place in the house at the most expensive price?"

"Shhh," Larry murmurs. "Let me handle this. He's staying here, right next to us, in the aisle. That still leaves plenty of room for people to come and go." As if it were a signal, we close ranks around Peter.

"I'm gonna get the police," the manager threatens, his enthusiasm for authority spent.

"Get them," says Larry.

"This is getting good," says Adam.

Peter says nothing. I pass the time by removing his jacket and stuffing it under his knees. That helps to tilt him backwards against the downward incline of the theater floor.

"Officer Rossi . . ." I smile, scanning his badge and extending my hand. It is the same tone of voice I use when I roll down the car window at a busy intersection to ask for directions. What else to a cop but disarming? "I'm Mary-Lou

Weisman. This is my husband, Larry, and our children, Adam"—giving him a tiny shove forward—"and Peter." I lift Peter's arm by the wrist so that he can shake hands with Officer Rossi.

The policeman takes Pete's hand in his. I watch his face change as he learns in a second not to expect a real shake back, not to expect more than the stir of something warm, small and sweet, something you would bring to your lips.

"What seems to be the problem?" He says his line with the bland impartiality that comes from repetitions like "Let me see your driver's license and registration," and the punctilious geniality of a conductor who must break the gentle to-and-fro rhythm of punching tickets and stop, swaying in place, to write a ticket and make change for a latecomer. Friend or enemy? I cannot read his face.

"This gentleman refuses to comply with the law and seat his child in the handicapped section," says the manager.

"Which is right there," I gesture, "behind the marble column, under the sound system."

"I'm sorry, madam, but I have to enforce the law," says the officer. The manager rocks back and forth on his heels.

"Don't be sorry. Just don't do it!" What am I doing recommending anarchy to a cop?

"If I make an exception for you, I'd have to make an exception for everyone," he chants, as if the answer were cranked out of him.

"No, you wouldn't!" I grab his sleeve. "You wouldn't. I'm not going to run down Broadway telling every paraplegic I meet, I promise." But I can tell from the way he is enduring me, his face standing at attention, that logic will not sway him.

I try another tack. "Peter has been waiting to see this show for months. How would you feel if he were your kid?" And I wonder if I mean "How would you feel if your kid had to sit behind a pillar?" or do I mean "How would you feel if your kid were so handicapped he couldn't shake hands?" and what the hell, why shouldn't I try to get some sympathy.

"Lady . . ." he pleads.

"If you think he should sit behind the pillar, Officer Rossi," says Larry, "you'll have to put him there yourself."

All eyes are on Officer Rossi. He taps his nightstick against his leg. He looks at his watch as if it holds the answer. He shakes his head slowly, trying to clear his mind.

"I can't do it," he says after a few moments. "I can't do it."

The audience has begun to clap with impatience.

"I'm not starting the show until he is in the handicapped seating," says the manager.

"We're not moving him," says Larry.

"I'll leave you folks to work this out," says Officer Rossi, beating a quick retreat.

"How would you like it if I was to get onstage and explain to the entire audience why they can't see the show?"

"That's not a bad idea," says Larry. "I'll tell you what. You go up and tell them your side of the problem, and then I'll go up and tell them mine. Then we'll invite them to vote. Very democratic. You and I will agree to abide by the audience's decision."

The manager stands doltish for a moment and then slouches down the aisle toward the stage and mounts the stairs. The audience quiets down to the sounds of hushes and starchy *Playbill*s folding closed.

"Damn it, Beatrice," I hear a woman stage-whisper to her companion, "don't tell me! We're going to get stuck with the understudy."

"Maybe he's just going to pass the hat for that damn actors' retirement fund, Edna."

"I hope you're right," says Beatrice.

"May I have your attention, please, ladies and gentlemen!" The manager holds his hands up in the traditional gesture. When quiet comes, he searches for some place to put them and places them one over the other, in front of his crotch. Then, thinking better of it, he plunges them into his jacket pockets and finally settles for joining them behind his back. "First, I'd like to apologize for the delay," he says, removing his hands from behind his back and pointing to his wristwatch as if he were going to talk in rebus. "It is due to circumstances beyond my control. A gentleman in the audience refuses to place his son, who's in a wheelchair, in the special handicapped area."

Shoulders pivot and fur coats slither over the wooden backs of rows of theater chairs, joined at the arms like paper cutouts, as the audience turns to identify the culprit. All eyes are on Peter.

"Now, I grant you," he continues when he regains their attention, "it's not the greatest seat in the house, but the kid'll get a good enough look, believe me. I like kids. I got three of my own. I want the kid should enjoy himself as much as the next guy, but we can't go around ripping out center-aisle seats—now, can we? We gotta have a place to sit too. A few years ago no theaters had seats for the handicapped. I grant you, that was bad. But now that we got 'em, they're not good enough. They want front row center. Whatcha gonna do?" He shrugs amiably. He is warming to the task. Now his hands lounge in his trouser pockets; his body is loose as he strolls stage right and stage left.

"Mr. Weisman—that's the gentleman's name—oughta respect the law, even if he doesn't seem to care how long he keeps you waiting to see the show that you paid your good money for. The fire law says in plain black and white that the aisles can't be obstructed by anything, including wheelchairs. That's about the size of it. It's not *my* law. It's the law of the state of New York. But Mr. Weisman doesn't like the law. So there won't be any further delay, we've worked out a deal. I tell you my side of the story, like I just did, and then he's gonna tell you his. Then you get to vote. Now, I'm assuming that you're law-abiding citizens like I am. I'm figuring you want to see the show and you want the kid to see the show too. So when Mr. Weisman gets done, I'm figuring you know how to vote and we'll get the show on the road.

Okay?" He ambles off, stage right, as cool as Hal Holbrook playing Mark Twain.

Larry moves quickly down the aisle. Defying perspective, he seems to grow larger as he approaches the apron. With his left hand on the lip of the stage, he hoists himself up with a single bound and turns to the audience. His jacket is askew; his necktie is caught on his shoulder as if he had just emerged from a wind tunnel.

"I'm Larry Weisman," he says simply, his arms hanging at his sides. "I drove up from Connecticut this afternoon with my wife and two sons—Adam, he's fourteen, and Peter, he's almost thirteen. Peter is in a wheelchair. We asked for and paid for four seats together, on the aisle. When we got here we discovered that Peter would have to sit apart from us in a special section for the handicapped. That special section was created by removing a single theater seat. The space created is located directly behind that marble pillar." He points and heads turn toward the spot he indicates. "The speakers for the sound system are mounted on the back of the pillar. The manager is correct. It is not the greatest seat in the house. It is, in fact, the worst seat in the house. I've suggested that Peter sit next to us in the aisle. I understand that's against the fire laws, but the fact is that since he can't drive without our help, the wheelchair is less of a hazard if we are nearby and can get Peter out in a hurry." He pauses for a moment. He seems reluctant to go, as if he had left something unsaid. He reaches out his hands for a second as if he were about to speak, and then lets them drop to his sides.

Say it, for Chrissakes, say it, Larry! I heckle him inside my head. Don't be such a tightass. You're turning the jury off. Tell them how he can't get into most restaurants. Tell them how he doesn't fit under most tables. Tell them how the children's room of the public library is at the top of thirty-six steps. Tell them how the kids at school tease him. Tell them how he used to be able to walk. Go ahead. Ask them how they would feel if it was their kid. Go ahead, ask them! Ask them how they would feel if it was their kid who was dying.

But he can't. Of course he can't.

Larry takes one more long look at the audience before he turns, his head low, and leaves quickly by the stairs, stage left.

"I blew it," he mutters as he sits down next to me. He drives his fist into his palm. "What the hell could I have said? I almost did it. I was tempted. I swear I almost did it. But at the last moment I couldn't. I just couldn't ..." He turns toward me, and I see tears in his eyes.

"I know," I whisper, taking his hand. "There's something worse than not getting what you want."

"They probably don't care, anyway," he says, so like a hurt child that I wonder that he doesn't notice it himself. "They don't care. They don't fucking care!" He sighs, "Oh, who knows, maybe if I were in their shoes, I wouldn't give a damn either."

"You would," I say, patting his hand. "You would. You're one of the nice people. You have a lousy temper, and you're stubborn, but you're very nice."

"Did you learn to make those subtle distinctions about human nature from your analysis?" he teases, squeezing my hand to say that he's all right now. "How's Pete taking all this?"

"I can't tell. I've been watching his face, but I can't tell."

The manager reappears on the center stage and raises his arms straight above his head, waving them from side to side, shaking his head, like a candidate humbled by his own charisma. "Okay, folks," he shouts above the upper respiratory cacophony unique to theater audiences, as if they, and not the performers, are about to be called upon to speak. "It's time to vote."

"Let the kid sit wherever he wants," sounds a man's voice from the balcony. It is the rallying cry.

"Let him sit in the aisle!" more voices shout.

Hands clap. The air rings with their ovation. Adam is clapping Peter's hands together. Peter is grinning from ear to ear. The tears from Larry's eyes escape and roll down his cheeks. My palms are stinging. The house lights dim.

In the fading light I turn to survey the scene and catch a glimpse of Officer Rossi leaning against an exit door. He is smiling.

"How do I know whether or not I want to go to camp if I've never been to camp so how can I know?" Peter is sitting at the kitchen table, drawing cars and drivers with no arms. "No arms indicates his sense of powerlessness," the school psychologist has noted.

"You've got a point," I answer, cutting the ends off the green beans. "I just have a feeling you'd have fun." I scramble to keep my voice light and casual. "Adam goes to camp, and he loves it."

"I'll go to Adam's camp."

I pause, almost enjoying the edge of the knife hard and thin and sharp against the meat of my thumb. "I wish you could, Pierre Ginzberg LaFarge." Oh, how I do. "Your camp will be as much fun for you as Adam's is for him." But I don't believe myself. "You'll do things you've never done before. They play a special kind of basketball and bowling and even baseball. Camp has an enormous heated indoor swimming pool. You can go swimming even in bad weather. That's better than home." I am a traitor, hellbent. I will defile my own nest, just to get him out of it. For me, goddamn it, for my sake, I will push him out, to sink or swim.

"Camp will be fun, a different kind of fun. A special kind. Besides, you'll meet a lot of nice kids." I remember the scant bifold brochure and the collage of black-and-white photos of children strewn like abandoned marionettes, in gleaming chrome wheelchairs, against a traditional camp background of pine trees, and I hope I am right.

"I think it's prejudice," says Peter.

"What's prejudice?"

"It's prejudice to have a special camp for handicapped kids. That's discrimination. Discrimination is against the

Constitution, and I think it's illegal, too."

"You've got a point, but I don't think there are any camps for both kinds of kids. Camp Robert is the best camp I could find for you." I wish the special camp for dystrophic children weren't called "Camp Robert." Did Robert live into his third decade, and did he know? Why couldn't they call it Camp Alpine, or Echo Lake or Vagabond or even Camp Wampawaramaug?

"Why does it have to have such a yucky name?"

"Probably because some yucky rich person gave them a lot of yucky money," I answer, fudging the truth.

"Do they know how to tuck me in at night? Do they know how to turn me? Will they hear me call, like you and Daddy?"

"Sure. They're used to taking care of kids. The counselors sleep in the same bunk with the kids. They'll hear you even better than Daddy and I."

Do they know, I wonder with an ache like homesickness, how to tuck a pillow between his legs when he's on his side so that his knees don't rub together and get sore? "Besides, I'll write them a note, explaining everything, telling them all about you." It'll take a bloody book. "And if I should forget anything, you can tell them yourself. Your mouth is in excellent working order. You could tell anyone how to care for you even if I didn't. You're very good at that."

"What if I miss you? What if I get housesick? Adam said he once got housesick."

"Homesick."

"Dogs get housesick, right?"

"Not quite. Dogs get housebroken." Like mommies, I think, discarding a withered bean.

"Your camp only lasts two weeks. I doubt if you'll have a chance to get homesick, although I think everyone would appreciate it if you'd stay housebroken."

"Can I bring my drums and my phonograph?" We're getting down to the nitty-gritty.

"Of course!"

"And wheelie?" His resistance is cracking.

"Absolutely. Wherever you go, wheelie goes."

"Okay, then, I'll go," he says reluctantly, "if you say so. But I still think they're prejudiced. Would you please get me a big piece of construction paper and my crayons?"

"How come you changed the subject?"

" 'Cause I'm done."

I take a few steps down the kitchen hall and open up the louvered doors of the play closet. I have won; so how come I feel so lost?

"I've decided to make a poster."

"Is it for school? An assignment?"

"Kind of."

I open up the box for him and spill out all the crayons near his right hand. As I am tucking one upper corner of the paper under his left hand, the telephone rings.

"Are you all set?" I feel the arbitrary urgency of the ring intrude on my nerves. "Do you have everything you need?" I hate it when Peter asks for things while I'm on the phone.

"Could I have some more apricots?"

"You're going to turn into an apricot." I grab a couple and stuff them into his waiting open mouth, noting that there really is such a thing as talking like a parent.

I reach for the phone and a cigarette. Time out. I hardly care who it is. I'll gladly listen to "This is Dolores" tell me about a freezer plan. "Hello?"

"Mrs. Weisman?"

"Yes." Thank God it's the right number. I sit down and put my feet up on the table.

"Oh, Mary-Lou? I didn't recognize your voice. This is Bob. Bob Lilienthal."

"Oh, hi, Bob." Bob and I are getting to be buddies, ever since Peter retaliated by running over Tony Pinelli's foot in school with his electric wheelchair, precipitating a parent-teacher conference on the uses and abuses of aggression, with satisfying results. "Well," Bob conceded at that time, "it sure solved the problem. We'll just let it go. Until he does it again. Then we'll probably let it go again." And we both laughed with surprised delight.

"I thought I ought to let you know," Bob says. "We're having a little trouble with Peter at school. I'm not sure how to handle it. I thought maybe you might have some ideas."

"What's the problem? Did he flunk another math test?"

"No," Bob answers. "We've solved that problem. I help him with the tests. We cheat. Nope, it's nothing that simple. Pete's on a hunger strike. He refuses to eat lunch at school. Today was the fourth day. I just thought you ought to know. He's angry because he was asked not to sit at a particular place in the cafeteria. Unfortunately, he and his friends like to eat lunch at a table near the food line. The wheels of his chair stick out into the line, and we're afraid that one of the children might trip and get injured."

"Did you explain that to Pete?" I glance at Peter. He is coloring intently, sliding his tongue slowly across his upper lip.

"I did, but you know Pete," Bob laughs. "He says he has a right to sit anywhere he wishes in the cafeteria. He says we're denying him his civil rights. He has the whole student body agitated and signing petitions—"

"He's passing out a petition?"

"I understand he has quite a few signatures. How do you suggest we handle this?"

"How about moving the food line?"

"That's easier said than done. It involves rearranging the whole traffic pattern in the cafeteria. The line is in the most logical, convenient place now."

"Well, I suppose you can just tough it out and see what happens."

"I thought you might be upset that Peter isn't eating lunch."

"Come to think of it, he's been eating bigger breakfasts lately, and more for snack when he comes home." I notice the depleted bag of apricots crumpled on the table. "I think he's taking pretty good care of himself."

"Well, then, if you don't mind, I think we'll tough it out, as you say. It's not so easy to move the food line."

"It may prove harder to move Peter."

"Why don't we wait and see what happens, so long as you don't mind about him not eating."

"I don't mind at all. Let me know what happens."

"Oh, I will, I will," Bob chuckles. "You know, I had him figured out all wrong at first. I thought he was just being a wise guy. Thirteen is a big age for wise guys. But not Pete. He's a wise guy, all right, but he really means business. I figured he'd last one day, maybe two. Frankly, I admire him."

"I do too. Thank you for saying so."

We say goodbye. I stand, hang up the phone, rest my hands against the warm receiver snug in its cradle and feel my heart lighten, feel a faint rustling, like feathers and the momentary weightlessness of lift-off.

"Was that Big Bad Bob Lilienthal calling you about the hunger strike?" Peter asks without looking up from his work.

"Yup."

"I'm glad you're not mad."

"Why should I be mad?"

"Well," says Pete, "I'm definitely being a pain in the ass. But what they're doing is unfair. I don't like being treated unfairly. I'm not going to let them get away with it, even if they are grownups, even if I do like them."

"How do the other handicapped kids feel?"

"I'm not sure. Some of them are with me, but some of them say they don't care. You know, there's a lot of prejudice in the world; it can be very discouraging," he goes on solemnly while I try to repress a smile at his dear banality. "There's so much prejudice that sometimes I don't know whether I'm being persecuted because I'm handicapped or because I'm Jewish."

I go over to him, laughing, throw my arms around his neck and give him big kisses. "I love you."

"I love you too," he says, as sweetly as a lover. "Since

you're not mad, I'll let you see my poster. I wasn't going to, but I need you to tape it onto the back of wheelie, anyway, so you'd find out, but now it doesn't matter because you don't mind, so you might as well look."

"May I look now?" I ask, making a big deal out of pressing my fingers against my eyelids.

"Okay. You can look."

All the letters are in capitals. Each is crayoned in a different color. Each letter is outlined in black. The letters get smaller and closer together, running downhill near the bottom of the paper:

WOULD YOU HAVE LET FRANKLIN DELAWARE ROOSEVELT SIT WHERE HE WANTED TO IN THIS CAFETERIA?

Peter's wheelchair stands empty at the shallow end of the pool near the stairs like a mute witness to a miracle, or evidence of a particularly dastardly crime.

Frail arms extended, bowed like a ballerina's embrace, Peter floats effortlessly, chest-deep, in the middle of the pool. "Like a cork," our amazed neighbors remark to me as if it were a compliment. Their macabre admiration is a stab in the gut. It is the same when they watch me lug him out of the water to place him back in his chair and they say "dead weight" before they wish they hadn't, eyes fixed on the ground, as if they'd just discovered something wonderful in the cracks of the flagstone.

But in the water he floats, as they say, like a cork. It's really quite apt. Couldn't be apter. His once dense muscles are nearly all turned to lighter, more porous fat. So he floats. Like a cork. The heaviest thing about him is his head, so he's always in danger. The tiniest wave can tip him over on his face. That's why I stand nearby in the pool, but not too nearby, not smotheringly nearby, arms outstretched, anticipating an emergency that always comes. Last summer the waves could not tip him over. This summer they can. That's progress—for the waves, I note, hating the irony but finding it irresistible.

I stare beneath the water's surface. I see the curve of his white buttocks, incandescent, and the concavity of the underside of his thighs where they have conformed, deformed, to a perpetual seated position. He sits in the water as he sits in his wheelchair, like a prisoner released from a tiger cage.

"Let's play bouncy-bouncy," says my fourteen-year-old son. Dark hairs grow from under his arms and around his penis, tiny tendrils like the finest of fine seaweed, soft and limp. And with no sense of irony whatsoever for this gallant young man in the body of a fetus, he adds, "And move your ass, woman."

"I am surrounded by chauvinist pigs and chauvinist piglets," I laugh, plowing furrows toward him with my arms, being careful not to disturb the water. I wrap his legs around my waist, and scooch a bit to fold his arms around my neck the way we did last summer. This summer his legs float away from my flanks, and his arms fall loosely from my shoulders.

"I'm not the man I used to be," Peter comments on the cruel defection of his limbs.

"It'll still work." I concentrate on the problem at hand. If I tuck his arms in between my chest and his, and if I hold him close and wrap my arms around his buttocks, to keep his legs in place, and use the flats of my hands against his lower back, it ought to work. It does.

"Bouncy, bouncy, bouncy!" we cry to the water. We bend down low and pop up high, and bend down low and pop up high, until Peter shifts in my arms and my thighs can no longer stand the strain.

"I'm exhausted," I confess, sputtering for air. I hold him in my arms, like a baby on the way to the changing table, grateful for the chance that water brings. I dance him around the pool, singing. "Ta-dump, ta-dump, ta-dump, dump-dump"—waltz, fox trot, even a tango—we cut through the water like sharks.

"Do it some more," Pete chortles in my arms. We twirl. I kiss his neck, his chest, his tummy, the tops of his knees. I hug him to me, cold skin against cold skin, repossessing every inch of this body I can never have on dry land. Such a treat! Such joy! We twirl some more in perfect happiness. I throw my head back, baring my neck to the heavens. If I can still hold him, God, then can't I still have him? Peter's head rests heavy on my shoulder. I'll make you a deal, God. Let me have him as long as I can hold him. Okay? Have we got a deal?

I pause a minute to give Him time to make up His mind. What He doesn't know is that I'm going to play a trick on Him. A real Rumpelstiltskin of a trick. He's going to be in-clined to make the deal, based on the fact that He knows I can hardly carry you now, and you're still growing. I'm not completely comfortable about fooling God, but if He can't understand that under certain extreme circumstances, any means is justified, then who can? If He says, "It's a deal," then, Peter, we're going to move South and stay in the water all day. We'll dance in our sky of blue and bounce as free as Chagall's bride and groom, floating past red donkeys and bouquets on their painted sea of blue sky. He'll never know until it's too late that he's made a Faustian bargain.

We twirl on, round and round, our mouths agape, our bodies drained of equilibrium. And then, if we get sick of water, we'll go to the moon. We're moon people, Peter. We're out-of-this-world, not-meant-for-this-planet moon people! You'll have to wear those lead-weighted shoes, but you won't mind. They won't feel heavy, the way your snow-suit jacket does, more each year. And there are no stairs. And everyone spills milk on the moon, Pete, and no one can cut his own meat. Oh, Petie! Let's fly to the moon!

"Stop, Mommy, stop! I'm too dizzy!" Peter calls madly from my arms. His head rolls crazily off my shoulder. "Help!" he yells just before his face threatens to sink beneath the surface.

"Don't worry!" I cry, grabbing him firmly around the shoulders and under the knees. "I've got you."

"Too bad we don't have a chandelier." Larry lopes around the bedroom lasciviously in his underpants. "Let's build a fire." He begins to remove the screen.

"Larry, it's June twenty-eighth. It's eighty fucking degrees. Who wants a fire?" I am sitting nude and cross-legged on the bedroom rug, frosting the inside of my diaphragm with Ortho-Gynol cream. The plump tube lies next to me.

"Just for atmosphere."

"I'm too hot."

"How about whipped cream? We've never tried whipped cream."

"Look, Larry. The kids are both away at camp for two whole weeks. Unless whipped cream dissolves rust, why don't we just do it plain and simple, until we both get the hang of it."

"I guess I just can't believe it. Two weeks. We can eat out!" he marvels, sitting down on the rug next to me.

"I can write all day if I want!"

"We can go to the movies!"

"And stay up late!"

"And sleep through the night!"

"And turn off the intercom!"

"And be alone with each other."

We take turns counting the ways.

"Heaven!" I swoon into his arms and lie there still for a moment, admiring his forearms as they rest on my belly.

"Piss me," says Larry.

"Shut up!" I giggle. "How did he seem to you when we dropped him off this morning. Did he seem scared?"

"Maybe a little. He was pretty quiet, but I think he's up to it. He's tough. You know Pete, he's never enthusiastic about anything ahead of time. By this evening he'll have organized a branch of the civil liberties union."

"I hope he'll be all right."

"I do too."

"Larry, did you notice how much further progressed the

disease seems to be in Peter compared to the other kids? There were kids Pete's age who were still walking. Peter's been in a wheelchair for *six years.*"

"Yeah, I noticed. Of course I noticed." He burrows his index finger deep into my bellybutton. "You're the inniest innie I ever saw."

"Do you think my thighs are getting flabby?" I pause, waiting for an answer. There is none. "I think they're beginning to look a little like cottage cheese, large-curd variety." I am still waiting for an answer. "Or maybe chiffon."

"I forget what I'm supposed to say." Larry shakes his head. "What are my lines? I can never remember my lines."

"You're supposed to say, 'Your thighs are gorgeous, Mary-Lou. They're not the least bit flabby.' "

" 'Your thighs are gorgeous, Mary-Lou. They're not the least bit flabby.' Hurry up and come to bed."

"Maybe a knee-lift would help." I place my hands on my thighs and jerk the skin upward. "I bet they do knee-lifts. If they can do eye pouches, they can do knees. I also think I may be getting Hadassah arm."

"What's Hadassah arm?"

"It's when your skin wiggles when you do like this," I demonstrate, raising my hand and diddling the flesh on the underside of my arm. "Later on it will actually swing. This is just an incipient case."

Larry runs his hands up and down my sides, molding my form as if he were sculpting it in sand. "You have such a beautiful body. For a woman of forty-one, you're incredible."

"How about for a woman of eighteen?"

Never enough. I can never get enough.

"You're insatiable."

"I just don't like getting older, Larry." I turn, shifting in his arms. "I don't think Dr. Tierney was right. I don't think Pete is going to live into his third decade. I don't think he's going to make it through his second." Larry doesn't say anything. "Sometimes I love him so much I want him to live forever, no matter what. I am willing, aching, to take care of him like this forever. I test myself. I imagine shaving his face. I imagine showing him films from the public library in his room—films on lion hunting in Africa and old Beatles reruns. I see us doing his homework from high school, even a correspondence course from college, if he should live that long. I test myself to see if I can stand it, and sometimes I can. And then sometimes I'm so tired and angry and sad that I wish he would die right now. I'm not sure for whose sake, his or mine."

There. I have said it. The words seem to lie scattered about us on the rug, like jagged glass.

"I know. I feel the same way. My fantasy is a little different from yours. I worry about his sexuality. I wonder about how we're going to handle that."

"I don't think he's going to live long enough for that to be a real problem."

We observe a moment of silence.

"I saw your father downtown at lunch yesterday. He went through his usual number about how he has been trying for weeks to find time to drop over to see the kids—"

"Spare me the details."

"He said something else. He asked me if we had ever considered institutionalizing Peter."

"Incredible! That's incredible!" I sit up with a jolt as if the world had just been born and I did not know the name of anything in it.

"Do you think it's incredible that he mentioned it?"

"No, not really. I don't think that's it," I think aloud, trying to understand why I am so shocked, so disoriented. "I suppose institutionalizing is really a pretty logical idea. An obvious idea. No. It's not incredible that he mentioned it. What's incredible is that we never thought of it. It just never occurred to me!"

"It never occurred to me, either. I suppose by the time we found out about Pete, the idea of an institution wasn't emotionally possible. Anyway, I'm sure he meant well. He's worried about you. He's worried that this is too much for you, especially now that Peter's so weak. He was just trying to be helpful."

"If he wants to be helpful, he can visit Peter more often." I pick at the pile of the rug. By the fifth yank, it dawns on me. "Did he mean we should think about institutionalizing Peter *now*?" I fairly shriek.

"I think he did."

"Oh my God!" Tears of rage and sorrow flood my eyes.

"I shouldn't have told you about it. I knew it would upset you. Look at us!" Larry takes his hands from my belly and gestures as if he were summing up the obvious to a jury. "Here we are, nude in the middle of the rug, alone together for the first time in years, with two beautiful weeks lying before us, and the first thing we do is bum ourselves out."

"You're right. And I started it too. I'll reform. Let's make a vow to set aside all sadness and anger for two weeks. Let's give ourselves a break. God knows we deserve it."

"Maybe God knows, but does He care? And, more to the point, does He give credit where credit is due?"

"I wouldn't count on it if I were you," I smile back. "The longer I live the more I begin to think that Grandma Perelmutter, Queen of the Yiddish Gypsies, wasn't so crazy, after all. It is all a matter of *mazel.*"

"Then what we need is a drastic change in *mazel.*"

I spring to my feet as if called on. "There'll ... be ... a"—I start off singing slowly, reaching for an imaginary straw hat and cane before I really get going—"change in the *mazel* and a change in the sea, dah-dah-dah-dah"—and now I'm really strutting my stuff, shaking my shoulders, lifting my legs like a trouper, waggling my hat—"and furthermore there'll be a change in me. My talk'll be different, my walk and my name, dah-dah-dah-dah, nothing about me's gonna be the—" Larry tackles me at the foot of the bed and we go sprawling.

Laughter is pierced by the ring of the phone.

"Hello?" Larry inquires jauntily, speaking into my left

breast, and then shifts his ear over to my right breast and pretends to be listening. The phone rings again. Still listening, Larry raises his eyebrows, makes a shocked "O" of his mouth, lays his hand over my left breast so that the phoner will not overhear, and whispers, "It's an obscene phone call. She wants to know if I have my panties on."

The phone rings again. "Go ahead, answer it for Chrissakes. Then we'll take it off the hook."

"Spoilsport," Larry mutters as he gets up, walks over and picks up the phone.

"This is he."

"If it's a client, get rid of him," I hiss.

Larry waves his hand impatiently in the air, as if trying to scatter the sound of my voice.

I sink back against the pillows and admire the armoring of muscle that keeps his thighs smooth, lean and hard. It's not fair.

"When did it happen?" Larry reaches for a pencil and a piece of paper. I try to read his face. Businesslike.

"Where?" he says. "Repeat that, please." He cradles the phone against his shoulder and writes. "We'll be right there. It'll take us a couple of hours. Tell him we're on our way." He replaces the phone gently in its cradle and picks his trousers up off the floor before he looks me in the eye.

"What is it, Larry?" I ask, but I must know. I am shaking so hard I hug myself around the knees to stop.

"It's Peter." Looking down, Larry steps into his trousers. "He broke his hip."

"On the first day of camp, Peter had an accident. It was a very silly accident. He bumped into a rock while speeding down a steep hill in his electric wheelchair, and he broke his hip. Now, hips take a long time to get better, and so Peter had to stay in bed, flat on his back, for twelve weeks ...!"

"I don't think I'm going to like this story," says Pete, his voice edged with anger and sorrow. "It's bumming me out even more."

"Be patient, Fudgetickle," Larry cajoles. "It's got a very happy ending; satisfaction guaranteed."

Larry is making up a story for Pete, as he does every night. I am standing at the kitchen counter, tearing up lettuce to go with the pizza, which lies on a rack in the preheated oven filling the air with the odor of pepperoni and hot prefabricated cardboard boxes. I look out through the screen door and onto the deck. Larry sits at Peter's bedside, his attaché case at his feet, his suit jacket thrown across the foot of the hospital bed.

Shadows cast by the large oak trees that surround the backyard deck dapple the silvery wooden planks. The deck seems to swim in the fading September light. The oak leaves, which opened in the spring, damp, wrinkled and glistening like a newborn's hands, now hang off the boughs limp, large and leathery, like boxers' gloves. Beyond, the pool glows a fluorescent, chemical green. Peter has been in bed for ten weeks. Two more to go.

Larry holds Peter's hand like a suitor and strokes stray wisps of hair off his damp forehead. I recognize the look, the moves. It has happened. At some moment, when I didn't notice, nor, perhaps, did he, it happened. He is changed. His face, once hard, arrogant and manly as a Roman coin, is as sad and soft as a madonna's, or a patriot's, and wise with dreadful knowledge. "All changed, changed utterly. A terrible beauty is born." The line of Yeats's appears across my brain, black and looped in spray-can script, like graffiti on a subway car. Love for Larry, love for Larry loving Peter fills my chest with tympanic fear and exaltation. Tears fill my eyes. We are lost. We are saved. For better or for worse, I have gotten my way.

"Ouch!" Peter complains testily. "The fucking acorns are falling on my head."

"Do you want me to wheel your bed back into your room?"

"No," Pete says. "I like to watch the squirrels."

"Well"—Larry lifts Peter's hand to his lips and turns it

gently to kiss his damp, wrinkled palm—"as I was saying before we were so rudely interrupted, hips take a long time to get better, and so Peter had to stay in bed, flat on his back, for twelve weeks! Now, twelve weeks is a long, long time. Twelve weeks is a lot of listening to Beatles records, a lot of drawing, a lot of eating, a lot of no swimming . . ."

"A lot of crumbs in my bellybutton . . ."

"And a lot of sponge baths . . ."

"And a lot of Pain and Strife of Family Life programs . . ."

"And a lot of reading . . ."

"And a lot of listening to Mommy sing her old camp songs . . ."

"And a lot of bedpans . . ."

"And a lot of boredom," Peter concludes their nightly responsive litany. I can feel that he is smiling, that he is no longer bored.

"Bor-ing! Bor-ing!" Larry and Peter howl in unison at the setting sun.

"Now, staying in bed for such a long time can be very boring. You can read for a while, watch TV for a while, play a game now and then, and talk to visitors when they come, but eventually, you get very bored."

"Bor-ing! Bor-ing!" They both break out again in a spontaneous chorus.

"But Peter was lucky because his bed could go out on the porch. His very smart mother saw to that the day the accident happened by sweet-talking a carpenter into breaking his bedroom wall down and installing a sliding glass door onto the deck."

"Mommy looked funny with a sledge hammer."

"At least you weren't bored that day," I holler from the kitchen.

"Peter could just lie on his back outdoors and watch the trees and the birds and the squirrels and the clouds.

"He noticed that the squirrels were particularly busy at certain times of the day. He figured out that those were their mealtimes. Suddenly there would be a lot of chattering. The branches over his bed would start to shake, and leaves and twigs and pieces of acorns would come tumbling down on the porch, all around Peter's bed. Sometimes they even landed on his head.

"And just as Peter watched the squirrels, the squirrels watched Peter. They were used to people, but most of the people they saw were moving very fast, either walking or running or on bikes or skateboards or in big scary cars. The squirrels were curious about people, but they were mostly scared of them.

"Peter was the first person the squirrels had ever seen who stayed so still for so long, just looking and smiling and singing and, once in a while, talking to them in a soft, friendly voice.

"The squirrels liked Peter and they chattered about him to each other. Word spread from tree to tree about this unusual person who was different from other people, and less scary.

"Finally, word reached the oldest, wisest, grayest squirrel of them all in his big hollow tree by the water, miles from where Peter lay. And when he heard about Peter, he said to the younger squirrels who were gathered around him, 'This is the perfect opportunity to lend the magic acorn. For years we squirrels have guarded the magic acorn, lending it from time to time to a human who was particularly deserving. As the oldest, wisest, grayest squirrel, I have the duty to decide whether this Peter is deserving and, if so, to lend him the magic acorn now that he is in need. We must leave at once for Peter's home so that I may observe him closely.'

"And so the old, wise, gray squirrel carefully placed the magic acorn in his mouth and scurried from branch to branch and from wire to wire, crossing roads and railroad tracks, until he reached the big oak tree which hung over Peter's deck.

"Peter had just come outside to get some sun. He was smiling and chattering just like a squirrel, and the old, wise, gray squirrel watched him very carefully, trying to decide if he was the right person to receive the magic acorn. He waited patiently until feeding time and then, while the other squirrels were leaping about, dropping pieces of their dinner on the porch near Peter, he aimed carefully and dropped the magic acorn right on his bed, next to his outstretched hand.

"The magic acorn was bigger and more perfectly shaped than other acorns. Its cap was tan and perfect and its bottom part was round and green with a sharp point at the end. It was a truly beautiful and special acorn.

"Peter picked it up and examined it carefully. Then he looked up at the tree where it had come from. He thought he saw a big, gray, old squirrel who seemed to be smiling. 'Thank you for the present, old squirrel,' said Peter. And at that moment the old, wise, gray squirrel knew he had done the right thing by giving the magic acorn to Peter.

"That night Pete slept better than ever before, with the magic acorn under his pillow. In the morning when he woke up, he felt terrific. He went out on the porch after breakfast and his new eighth-grade teacher came to visit and stayed for lunch. Lunch was a tuna-salad sandwich, which Peter didn't really like.

" 'I wish I had a pizza instead of this yucky sandwich,' Pete said. And just then there was a puff of white smoke and a flash of light, and there on the plate, where the sandwich had been, was a pepperoni pizza.

" 'How did you do that?' Peter's teacher asked.

" 'I didn't do it. It just happened,' said Peter.

"Peter had forgotten all about the acorn under his pillow. And even if he had remembered it, he wouldn't have thought it had anything to do with changing the tuna-fish sandwich into a pizza because he didn't know that the acorn was magic.

"The days went by and stranger and stranger things kept happening. People Peter wanted to see would suddenly show up, just because Peter happened to be thinking about them.

And most wonderful of all, Peter's hip got better right on time, and he hardly missed any school.

"Once Peter got out of bed and back into his electric wheelie, of course he forgot all about the acorn. It sat, unnoticed, on the window sill in his room.

"The magical, mysterious things stopped happening, but that was okay. Peter was happy and he didn't need any magic now that his hip was all better.

"Then one night late in September, while Peter was fast asleep, he dreamed that a big gray squirrel came in his window and stood by his pillow for a long time, looking at him, and then that he left by the open window, with something in his mouth."

"That's a good story," says Peter after a little while, and then he adds, "Do you believe in magic?"

Thin ice. We are on thin ice. The neural alarm goes off in my head.

"What about *you*, Fudgetickle?" Larry turns the question. "Do you believe in magic?"

"I believe in it," Peter answers softly, "but I don't count on it."

"Here, then!" Larry presses an acorn into Peter's hand and folds his fingers closed around it. "You hang on to this; it's the one that klunked you on the head. I'm going to change my clothes for dinner. I'll be back in a minute to keep you cumps. As soon as Adam gets home, we'll all eat dinner with you out here on the deck." Larry closes the door and calls back through the screen. "By the way, is Dumps coming to dinner tonight?"

"Nope, she can't," Pete answers. "She's too busy. The magazine goes to press tomorrow morning. She's going to come tomorrow night after work, with Suka."

Dumps. I smile over a bowlful of tattered iceberg. Dumps. From Prudence. Prudumps. Dumps. From among casual acquaintances, Peter chooses our friends, and from the best of them, names a family. He calls them our "fake family." Fake Aunt Gloria and Fake Aunt Shelley. Pretend sister Therese.

Big brother John. Uncle Kenny and Patsy-O. The Humdingers. Doug and Spoonbread Annie. Crazy Uncle Milton and Matt and Mitch. They are related by Peter.

We even have a family dog, Suka, who prances about the house with Peter's slippers in her mouth, as authentically all-American and boy's-best-friendly as if she bounded out of a Norman Rockwell print.

"What are we having for dinner?" I hear Pete call from the deck.

"I think it's tuna salad," Larry answers, giving me a wink as he passes through the kitchen. "You'll have to ask Mommy."

"What are we having for dinner?" Pete shouts bravely into the kitchen. "I hope it isn't tuna salad."

"No," I call back as nonchalantly as possible, "it's pepperoni pizza."

"Larry!" I nudge him in the arm. "Wake up. There's something wrong."

"Wassamatter," Larry mumbles, turning in his sleep.

"There are funny sounds coming over the intercom."

"Maybe Peter's talking in his sleep." Larry raises his head off the pillow just long enough to catch a glimpse of the illuminated face of the clock radio on his bedside table. "Shit! It's only five A.M."

"No, listen! It sounds as if he's talking *with* someone." I reach over and turn up the volume knob. In between its usual, punishing squawks we hear:

"Shove over, I'm coming in."

"Okay, but first move me over. Hey, careful, my hip still has a week to go. First take away the pillow that's leaning against me and roll me over on my back. That's it. Now take the pillow that was between my legs and put it behind my knees. That's good. Now fix my arms. I want them at my sides. I don't want to hold Soft Gray right now. Put him on the bureau. Perfect. Now one more thing. Pick up my head and turn over my pillow; this side is all covered with drool-ies. Thanks. Now crawl over me and get in. Oops. I forgot one thing. Just lean over me—the controls are on my side—and push the button that says 'head up.' "

The sound of Pete's new hospital bed hums through the intercom like science fiction. "Okay. That's high enough. Thanks. What are you doing here so early in the morning, Dumps?"

"I just had to get out of where I was. I'm sorry if I woke you up. I'll just snuggle in here with you, pull the covers up over my head and die."

"Ouch!" Pete cries. "Your elbow is digging into my ribs; it's pointy."

"Sorry, darlin'." Prudence's muffled voice meanders through the dry walls and into our waiting ears. "I can't do anything right today."

"Maybe you got out of the wrong side of the bed."

"Nope. Just out of the wrong bed altogether."

"Dumps! Yuk! Do I smell liquor on your breath? Are you sauced?"

" 'Yes,' you smell liquor on your breath, and 'no,' I'm not sauced," Prudence confesses in her wanna-make-something-of-it? tone. "I *was* sauced. Now I'm just hung over. I'm also disgusting."

"Poor Dumps. You sound sad."

"I'm not sad. I'm pissed."

After a few seconds of electronic silence, we hear a whisper through the wires. "Okay. So I'm sad."

"That's bad. Tell me what happened and I'll fix it."

"Promise not to tell your mother if I tell you? She'd really be furious at me if she knew. She'd give me one of her big lectures, and I'm definitely not in the mood."

"I promise not to tell."

"Uh-oh," Pru remembers darkly, like a child, "the last secret I told you, you told Adam, and Adam told Therese, and Therese told John, and John told Uncle Kenny, which resulted in there being no Häagen-Dazs rum raisin *pour moi.*"

"That's because it was about food. I can keep secrets if they're not about food. Come out from under the covers and tell me. Turn my head to the left a little. A little more. Perfect. Now tell me."

"I'm ashamed. I'm weak. I'm so goddamn weak I don't believe it."

"What did you do, Dumps?"

"Remember that asshole I brought over a few weeks ago to meet you, the guy you said wasn't good enough for me, the guy I supposedly broke up with two weeks ago?"

"You mean Kumquat Head?"

"You got it."

"Oh Jeezus, Larry." I lean over and turn up the volume on the intercom. "I think Dumps went back to Kumquat Head. That *creep*! How could she *do* it?"

"I was at a party last night. Toward the end, when people were beginning to go home, I started to feel lonely. I had no one to go home to, no one to go home with . . ."

"Poor Dumps."

"Don't get me wrong. I don't want to be married or anything like that. The last thing I want is to end up leaning on someone. Just an occasional warm, loving experience will do. So I got into the car, drove over to Kumquat's house and . . . now I hate myself."

"What for?"

"For being so fucking weak and needy. For being one of the *New York Times'* hundred neediest cases."

After a moment Peter asks, "Is it bad to need someone?"

The intercom is silent again, except for the uninterrupted, tiny scream, as high and thin as a wire, that lets us know it's turned on. Prudence doesn't answer.

"Don't be sad, Dumps." Peter breaks the silence. "Someday you're going to find a good man you can lean on."

"I already have one, Petie. You."

"Pick up my hands and put them around your neck and hold them there so I can hug you. That's right. Good. Now turn your head, put your cheek right up against my mouth

and relax so I can give you one of my special suction kisses."
A long slurp, followed by a loud pop, resounds through the
intercom. "I love you, Dumps."

"I love you too."

"Do you think the age difference is too great? I'll be fourteen on November second. When's yours?"

"I'll be forty-one on December fourth. Shit."

"You're a little bit younger than my mother; still, we'd
better hurry up and get married. I'm not allowed to marry
her. She says it's against the rules. Are there any laws against
marrying fake relatives?"

"I don't think so."

"Great! Then we can do it," says Peter.

"You've got a deal," says Pru.

"Will you do me a favor, Dumps?"

"Sure, darlin'."

"Piss me."

"Please unplug my wheelie and bring it next to the bed."

"*Oui, mon capitaine,*" says Larry, saluting smartly and turning to obey. "Hup, two, three, four. Hup, two, three, four."
About-facing at the door, he marches on toward the living
room.

Today's the day Peter gets out of bed. His hip is healed.
I've pushed the "head up" button so that the mattress is
tilted as far as it can, holding Peter in an oblique version of a
seated position. The covers, usually held straight across his
chest by being tucked under his arms, have slipped downward with gravity and gathered just below his waist, where
the bed has bent him, revealing the paunch of fat that gir-
dles his middle. I notice the contours of his legs beneath the
blanket, bowed, from top to toe, like a pair of parentheses.

His arms have never really had any shape. The tri- and
bi-ceps were devoured even as they developed. Like the arms
of a starving person, his are widest at the elbow. They rest at
his sides.

As I study the barely perceptible rise and fall of his chest, his skin seems translucent. I imagine I can see his lungs and his heart, as if he were an X-ray.

His embryo head, so too big, so dark around the eyes, topples from his stem-thin neck and slips toward his meager shoulder.

"Here, Petie; let me straighten you out." I tuck a pillow behind his head and step back from the bed.

I wonder how old he is, his real age, this mutant life, this doomed experiment, my aged baby. Is there some formula, some way to calculate, some number to multiply by 7 perhaps, like dog-years by people-years; or maybe some number to divide by, the way you figure out a Manhattan address to the nearest cross street.

Larry appears at the bedroom doorway. "Your chair awaits, sir."

"Does it still work after all these weeks?"

"It sure does." Larry pushes the lever that engages the two motors, flips the toggle switch to "on" and presses the joy stick. The chair bolts forward.

"Okay," Peter presides. "Now turn it off and lock the brakes."

"Chair, off. Brakes, on," Larry reports.

"Is my posturepedic contour shell firmly in place? Are the wings attached?"

"Posturepedic contour shell firmly in place; wings, likewise," Larry assures him, making an imaginary adjustment to the polyurethane seat and back rest, which have been molded to accommodate the curvature of his spine, his scoliosis, and the foam pads that protrude from each side and fit snugly under his armpits. Peter can no longer sit in his chair supporting his own weight. He hangs.

Respiratory function. Osteoporosis. Scoliosis. Breathing. Brittle bones. Hunchback. I am learning to appreciate the euphemisms of medicine. "Everything is in readiness, sir, awaiting your further orders." Larry clicks his heels.

There is a pause. "Are you sure you can still lift me?"

"Positive." Larry flexes his muscles. "Let's go!"

"No!" Peter's voice is sharp.

"What's the matter?" Larry asks.

"I'm scared it's going to hurt."

"I don't think it's going to hurt, Pete," I try to reassure him. "You're probably a little stiff, maybe a few kinks to shake out, but it shouldn't hurt." I reach toward him to lift his leg, to bend it at the knee, to show it doesn't hurt.

"Don't touch me, don't touch me!" Peter shrieks and his eyes widen with alarm.

"Stop that! Stop that! There's nothing to be scared of," Larry says in his calm, confident voice, the one he uses for taking Peter up escalators backwards in his wheelchair.

"Don't touch me, don't touch me, don't touch me!" Peter shrieks over and over again. His head thrashes. His eyes, though wide open, look blind, as if he were staring into himself. I shoot a look at Larry, my heart pounding. Peter has never been out of control before.

"Janis Joplin! Jimi Hendrix! Jim Morrison," Peter shrieks as if he were seeing a ghost. It's crazy. It must be a joke. It's like an act, like someone acting hysterical. I don't know what to do.

"What does it mean, Larry?"

"Janis Joplin's a rock singer," says Larry above Peter's screams.

"Janis Joplin! Jimi Hendrix! Jim Morrison!" Now the screams come faster, in terrified, staccato yelps, as if someone were shaking him violently by the shoulders. His head whips back and forth on his slim white neck. I can't believe he has such strength.

"They're all rock stars," says Larry. "And they're all dead. Drug overdoses, I think."

"But why? What does it mean? I don't know what they mean!" I cry, and then, suddenly, I do. That's the face that death wears when you're fourteen years old in America in 1978 and you love rock music.

I fling myself belly down on the bed on top of Peter, letting him feel my weight. I hold the sides of his rigid head tightly in my hands, press my cheek to his cheek, hard. "Shoo, baby, shoo, baby, shoo, shoo, shoo," I chant, over and over again.

"I'm scared, I'm scared, I'm scared!" he shouts, staccato and shrill, while I hold on, rocking his body to and fro with mine, wrestling for his soul.

"Shoo, baby, shoo, baby, shoo, shoo, shoo," I whisper, loudly, insistently, then louder still, rocking and chanting, rocking and chanting, until my voice captures, overpowers and subdues the frantic rhythms of his cries.

"Better?" I whisper softly in his ear. He does not speak, but his eyes look clear and his thrashing head rolls to rest between my hands. Slowly, gently, I roll off of him, sit on the edge of the bed and take his small, limp hands in mine.

The bogey man has struck at last, in spite of the night light and checking under the bed and peeking into the closet and behind the drapes. That villain, who for years has menaced the edges of Peter's world, hovering in corners, casting fearful shadows even in the broad daylight of his youth and innocence, has lowered the black cape from in front of his eyes and revealed himself. And I know I cannot dance him away, or sing him away, or joke him away, or even love him away. Not for long.

"I understand" are the only words of communion I can find for the terrible knowledge that has just invaded his soul. "I understand," I repeat, looking steadily into his eyes, hoping I will not flinch.

"I really freaked out, didn't I?" says Peter, returning to normal.

"One of the finest freak-outs I've ever seen," says Larry, bending over to give him a kiss. "Are you ready to get up?"

"Not quite."

"I think I'd freak out too," I allow, "if I'd been in bed for three months, wanting to get up, but forgetting what 'up' even feels like. It's going to feel good, Petie. You're going to be glad you got up. You've just got to push through this scared place. Maybe if I wiggle your body a little, you'll see that you're in working order.

"Wiggle his little toes," I cackle like a silly witch, running to the foot of the bed to wiggle toes that cannot wiggle on their own.

"Wiggle his floppy ear," Larry joins in at the head of the bed.

Peter smiles indulgently. It's working.

"Hello legs!" I carry on, sliding my arms behind his knees and waggling them up and down. "And hello shoulders!" I cry, cupping them in my palms. They accommodate so flexibly. He is literally falling apart. "And for the piece of resistance—hello hips!" I slide my hands beneath his buttocks and jiggle gently, very gently.

"That didn't hurt." Peter smiles a brave smile.

"Are you ready now?" I ask, giving his hips one more jiggle.

"Just one more thing," says Peter. "Would you please take the mirror off the wall?"

"Sure."

Wondering why, I remove the mirror from over his bureau, realizing as I do that the only reflection I have ever seen in it is my own, choosing his clothing from the drawers.

"Push 'head down,' and roll me over on my side, Dad."

Larry presses the button, and we watch while the bed slowly unfolds Peter to horizontal. Then, surely and swiftly, in the psychological tradition of Band-Aid removal, Larry flips him onto his side.

"Now what?" I ask, feeling the weight of the mirror in my arms.

"Well, I've been thinking . . . ever since I've been in a wheelchair, ever since I couldn't walk anymore, I've never seen the back of me. Other people see the backs of themselves all the time, any time they want to . . ."

"So you want to see the back of you?" I ask, moving toward him with the mirror.

"Actually," he admits, "what I really want to see is my ass."

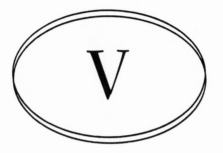

Breathe, damn it, breathe!

The thin black needle on the respirator dial swings to the right. It arcs at the number 32 before it slips back to zero. I hold my breath and keep watching. The needle swings again, reaching 32 before it falls back. Peter breathes.

Beat, damn it, beat!

The orange digital numbers on the cardiac monitor readout screen oscillate perpetually, blinking 122, 123, 122. The heartbeat of sleep. Peter sleeps.

Nurses laugh over Styrofoam cups in the lounge. The digital numbers blink 117. Peter wakes, but just for a moment; 122, 123, 122—he sleeps again.

I sit by your bedside, watching you live. You are far away from me. Farther than sleep. Farther, much farther, than the stretch of turnpike that led us here, breaking through the wooden arm at the tollgate, bells ringing, the accelerator gunned to the floor—"Mommy, I can't breathe!"—farther away still when hands grabbed you from me in the emergency room. "Suction! Suction! Lady, get out of the way, please." Even farther into your nightmare ("Mommy's here! Mommy's here!") you slip, eyes rolling, neck heaving, as they plunge a plastic tube down your throat ("Cough!") drawing it up and down ("Cough!") sucking at the mucus in your throat. But you cannot cough, not even a little.

I cough. I gag. I hold my mouth wide open for you. This is as far as I can go. But it's no good. You are gone. A rubber-gloved hand throws the suction tube aside. "Get the respirator; I'll bag him. *Move,* lady, *please."*

"Here's Soft Gray. Soft Gray is going with you!" I cry, as far away you go, rolling down the hall in a litter, out of my sight, while someone I do not know runs alongside, squeezing life into you from a black rubber bladder.

Now I am a visitor. A relative. A mother with a white pass.

"His mother to see Peter Weisman," says the volunteer in the waiting room into the special phone that connects with the nurses' station in the intensive care unit. "You may go in."

Does this straight corridor lead back to you? Is this time just a grim detour in the circle of love? Or is the earth flat, and beyond here "there be dragons"? I press the square metal button on the wall—"Stanley Magic Door Press to Operate"—and the double doors that lead to ICU swing open. I see you. There, behind the half-drawn muslin curtain, I see you.

"Weisman, Peter 100722" says the plastic bracelet around your wrist. No little baby-boy blue-and-white beads this time. A few inches above, 5% saline and dextrose drips through a plastic tube and into a hollow needle inserted in your vein. Two milky-white spiral hoses meet at a stiff plastic tube that grows from your mouth, held in place with a gag of adhesive tape. Only the corners of your mouth show, pink and wet with unswallowable saliva. I follow where the two flexible tubes lead, across your chest, off the side of the bed, one gurgling air into a container of water, the other into the respirator.

Black wires, grounded in white rubber suction cups affixed to your chest, tangle about your neck and shoulders before they plug into the cardiac monitor, mounted high on the wall above the respirator.

I stand up and tentatively draw back the sheet. Your penis is sheathed in a condom catheter; urine has collected in amber segments inside the clear plastic tube where it coils on the bed near your knees.

So far away, I cannot find a place to kiss you. Gingerly, I bend over you, like a stranger, and touch my lips to your cool, cool forehead.

The respirator hisses, the sound of air escaping from the unpinched neck of a balloon. The needle swings. Your chest rises and falls.

I reach toward the foot of the bed for Soft Gray and sit back down in the visitor's chair. I press my face into his woolly belly and greedily breathe in the scent of you—baby talc, stale sweat, and the cloying adolescent juices of glands overflowing with new life—and enjoy the taunting, sweet, rich musk of years of nights spent in your arms.

Oh, Pete, I'm sorry. Please forgive me. If I was wrong not to tell you, I'm sorry. If you had asked, I would have told. But you didn't ask the question, and I didn't tell the answer, not when you went into a wheelchair, not when you could no longer propel the wheels by hand and we bought you a motorized chair, not when we switched from No. 2 Venus Velvets to No. 1, not when you accepted a flexible straw instead of picking up your milk glass, not when each summer proved you could swim less than the summer before, until you could only float; not once, not ever, did you ask the question. Not once, not ever, did you let on that you knew the answer. But I heard all the questions you never asked. Did you hear all the answers I never spoke? Was it our little secret, our little game? Did you go into this with your eyes wide closed? Or, dear God, have I betrayed you?

I really didn't know what was right. I still don't even now. Even now that the jig is nearly up, and there are no more tricks left but the respirator, I want a miracle. I want you to live. I want you back, for as long as you can stay. But you have to know, Petie, I have no more tricks left. Or do you know that, too?

Now I have a question for you to answer. Do you want to live? There's a green rubber plug on the wall, just a few feet away. I'll pull it if you say so. I think I have the nerve. I hope I do. But it's not my decision this time; it's yours. You have to decide if it's worth the fight. Even if you win this time, you'll be back. Or do you know that, too? You decide. This time, it's up to you.

I stand up and gently lift your right wrist, trailing its intravenous tube, and tuck Soft Gray into the crook of your arm. The digital numbers blink 117, 117, 117, 117. You are awake. Your eyes open.

I smile, for all I'm worth, into your face, across the white sheets, past the tubes and the wires, the strange hands, the turnpike and the tollbooth. "Hi, Fudgetickle Entworth LaRue. It's Mommy. I love you."

The corners of your mouth struggle to turn upward against the downward tug of the adhesive tape, and light glistens in the tears of your eyes.

"Okay, then, petunia puss," I whisper, crawling into the bed. "Let's see how fast we can get the hell out of here."

"Throat hurts terribly?" Holding the clipboard under the light at the head of the bed, I read Peter's chicken-scratch message back to him.

"Yes," he blinks emphatically and then opens his eyes wide. We have worked out a code. Big blink, wide open, means "yes," because nodding hurts. Moving his head from side to side means "no." Side to side doesn't hurt. Holding his hand delicately at the wrist, I place the liquid-flow ballpoint pen between his fingers and follow his almost imperceptible lead like a robot while he carefully, exhaustingly, writes his message. That nod, that blink, that wobbly print are the only life lines we've got. The plastic hoses do the rest.

"You know, Pockie, you don't have to write 'Throat hurts terribly' when it's so difficult to print clearly at this angle. Why don't you just write 'Throat'; I'll know what it means."

Peter blinks his eyes in rapid succession, signaling a message to communicate. I prop the clipboard on his stomach with one hand and take his wrist with the other. *"How ... else ... can ... I ... complain?"* writes the moving hand, taking special care with the question mark.

I smile, take the clipboard, and write in big, bold print: *"Fuck! Shit! Milk! Cookies!"* "Remember, Pete?"

The corners of his mouth turn up, spilling a thin rivulet of saliva down his chin. I reach for a tissue, before he has a chance to blink me to attention.

"It's just spit," I say, dabbing at his chin. "Terrific stuff, spit. I'm crazy about it." A glare from Peter lets me know I'm overdoing it. "I'll get some Xylocaine from the nurse."

I push aside the muslin curtain, which travels swiftly and soundlessly on a round-cornered metal track in the plaster ceiling, and step toward the nurses' station—control center—located dead center in the huge, square room. The nurses huddle there in a circle, like voyeurs, before the screens numbered one through ten, tending their patients, adjusting the volume and fine tuning. The machines inhale and exhale, blink, twitch, sleep and cry out in alarm.

Behind the nurses' backs, the patients, plastic tubes down their throats, expand and contract under their sheets like bagpipes playing the music of technology.

These machines are real, more real than the adjacent lives they obscure and serve, the objects of their attention, lying small and silent under the sheets. Here life is perpetually guaranteed if only they will have it. Here, if death were infectious, it could sneak so easily past the nurses while their backs are turned, and slip so easily through the muslin curtains that line all four walls, separating, isolating the human conditions, and join them together at last.

Here there is no color but white, no light but the gleam of steel and glass and the gaudy flash of digital numbers, no sound but the metronomic beat of a mechanical pulse and the hiss of the respirators' bellows; no smell but the heavy, sweet stench of infection. The room fights for its life.

What's wrong with this picture is me again. Dungarees amid white nylon uniforms. An English major who cannot balance her checkbook because she cannot understand why a nine in the tens column doesn't mind being borrowed from and reduced to an eight, so that the two in the ones column can become a three that you can take another three away from—a humanist, dropped like a fifth column behind the enemy lines of science and technology. An alien, a mother, irrelevant, at best a bother, at worst a threat, to be tolerated on doctor's orders, but only up to a point.

"Ahem." I try to get their attention. "Ahem."

"Yes?" She turns to look at me, her lips set in a "what— you again?" smirk. It's Nurse C. Bocanfusco. She wears her scissors clamped on her hip.

"Peter's throat is hurting him a lot. Could he have some of that—what do you call it . . . oh, yes—Xylocaine?" I prostrate myself to the point of acting stupid, so as not to threaten their authority.

She consults the chart. "He's not due for more Xylocaine for another two hours."

"He really needs it; he's experiencing considerable discomfort." Pain is not permitted on this floor. I am catching on to the lingo. "Considerable discomfort," as in, "Mr. Wisznicki in number six is experiencing considerable discomfort."

"He's not due for two more hours," she repeats.

Okay. No more Mr. Nice Guy. "Look"—and my hands go on my hips—"unless it's really bad for him to have Xylocaine more frequently than you have it down on your chart, I don't see why he can't have it. For God's sake, the kid's had a pipe down his throat for three days now!"

"He ought to be used to it by now."

"*Used* to it! Unless you've had a pipe down your throat for three days, I don't think you are in a position to comment on how much pain my son is experiencing."

Her face contracts at the mention of the word.

"Mrs. Weisman, I have other patients to attend to right now. I'll give Peter some Xylocaine as soon as I'm finished."

"How long will that be?"

"A few minutes. He can wait a few minutes."

"I don't see why he should. Are you afraid you're going to spoil him? I'll give him the Xylocaine. I know how to do it. You just insert the hypodermic needle in the top and draw out the plunger to four whatevers, and then you just squirt it down his throat."

"We can't permit mothers to medicate their children."

"Why not? I've been doing it for fifteen years." I try another tack. "Look, you're overworked. I can tell. Why not let me do what I can safely do for Peter? That way I won't have to keep bothering you for things I can do myself."

"We cannot make an exception in your case."

"Why not? Are you afraid I'm going to abuse the privilege and run around the unit shooting people up with Xylocaine? Jeezus!"

"Mrs. Weisman, as it is, you have stayed here long past visiting time. I think you should leave now. You may come back for ten minutes out of each hour. Those are the rules."

I don't have to decide whether or not to leave. I'm just not leaving. I can tell by the way my feet suddenly seem rooted in the vinyl floor. "I'm not leaving, and either you're going to give Peter the Xylocaine right now or I am."

Without speaking, she steps back into the nurses' station, gets the Xylocaine and walks toward Pete's cubicle. I follow.

"All right, Peter, I'm going to give you some Xylocaine to relieve the discomfort in your throat," she shouts toward him, without actually looking at him. Deftly, she squirts the painkiller down his throat and drops the spent syringe in the wastepaper basket. "Better?" she yells, turning to leave.

On her way out she pauses to inspect the collection of stuff on the table at the foot of his bed; a bell, the kind you find on the counter of a delicatessen, so that he can call a nurse with the flat of his hand if I'm not around—his fingers are not strong enough to depress the call button—and the clipboard. Soft Gray Hippo, who gets in the way of the wires, is wedged into the grappling hook that hangs above the bed from the ceiling, dangling IV bags.

"Get rid of the hippo," she says, drawing the curtain closed behind her.

"The hippo stays," I say after her. "The nurses are a pain in the ass," I complain to Peter, before I realize that's wrong. He's got to trust them. I can't be there all the time. I can't be there at night. "Actually, they're perfectly nice. It's just that they get hassled. It's very difficult to take care of so many sick people at once."

Peter blinks rapidly. I reach for the clipboard. *"Why . . . do . . . they . . . hate . . . me . . . ?"* he writes, his eyes searching my face.

"Hate you? Who could hate you? They love you. Everybody loves you. You are the world's most irresistibly lovable person. You are the most edible, mungible, fungible, extraordinarily burunctious, glumdideous flopnick in captivity. Besides that," I finish, giving his ear lobe a lick, "you're nice."

But deep down I sense that he is right. They do hate him. And they hate me, too.

"It's going to take a miracle," Dr. Braverman whispers, shaking his head sadly from side to side. "I don't know. It all depends on whether the virus he's got responds to any of the antibiotics we're giving him. Assuming, of course, that his heart holds up. It should; it's strong."

We are standing at the X-ray viewer located just outside of Peter's curtained cubicle in intensive care. Dr. Braverman slips the upper corners of the latest chest X-ray under the black metal tabs and flips the toggle switch to "on." Peter's tadpole torso swims into view. His extravagantly arched ribs are stretched thin and opened wide, as if pleading for mercy for his laboring lungs and faltering diaphragm.

"You can see the pneumonia; here"—he points to a shadowy mass, like a storm cloud, at the bottom of one lung—"and here. It spread to the left lung yesterday."

"Then he's getting worse?"

"I can't be sure. There's no difference between today's and yesterday's X-ray. That may mean he's holding. There's no way we can know except to wait and see which way it goes. It's been six days. We've got to worry about the next step."

"What next step?" If I can't have comfort, I will settle for clarity.

"We have to begin to wean him from the respirator—today."

"Wean"; I remember "wean," the tugging ache, so near to pleasure, of letdown, the surge of milk rushing from glands to nipples. I was sitting next to Larry in Alice Tully Hall. David Oistrakh held his violin high. The encore was a Paganini "Caprice." He attacked it with his bow. Letdown. My lap felt damp. Two stains grew on my navy blue dress. I looked at my wristwatch. Feeding time. I nudged Larry, tapped my watch and grimaced with a mixture of horror and delight at the bovine wonder of me.

"Here I am in Alice Tully Hall," I whispered, "pumping out all this good stuff, and Peter's back home in the arms of the baby-sitter, happily sucking Enfamil."

"Moo," Larry whispered, giving me a big smile. He lifted my hand to his lips, kissed it softly and held it in his lap until the "Caprice" was over.

"How can you wean him from the respirator when he's got pneumonia in both lungs?" I raise my voice. Dr. Braverman moves the flats of his hands up and down, like a conductor, to shush me.

"It's not a matter of 'how,' " he whispers. "We have no choice. We must begin to wean him today."

"But why? Why not wait until he's better?"

"Because he's got to be off the respirator entirely at the end of two weeks, that's the pediatric maximum. After that, there's too great a risk of infection from the tube. We've got eight days left in which to wean him. The problem is, he doesn't meet any of the parameters for weaning. Not a single one. And yet, we've got to do it. Otherwise . . ."

"Otherwise what?"

"Otherwise, we'll have to do a tracheotomy. We'll have to cut a hole in his trachea and keep him on the respirator until he's ready."

"I won't let you do that. He's had enough. Too much."

"I know. It's going to take a miracle to get him off this respirator in eight more days. But if he can't do it, we will perform a tracheotomy. You'll have to let us. I believe we can save his life this time."

"You doubt you can do it again?"

He shakes his head to confirm my worst fears. "Next time, I would advise you not to let us put him on a respirator."

I stand at the edge of reason and understanding, mute and bewildered, out of questions, out of answers, out of control.

"Let's not worry about that until we have to. How's Pete's mood?"

"Not so good. The first three days he was really incredible—brave, positive, easy to amuse, looking forward to seeing Adam and Larry—and now I can't make him smile. He's even stopped being nasty."

"That's not good." Dr. Braverman looks at the tops of his shoes. "But I'm not surprised. This is no place for a kid."

"The Gestalt around here stinks. It doesn't have to be as awful as they make it. There was no reason to make me take Soft Gray home. That was just plain mean. Peter notices it too. They're always trying to throw me out. I just don't leave. It's like war, the worst kind of war—very civilized."

"I'll see what I can do about it. Peter's going to need everything he can get on his side. He's going to have to fight to get off the respirator. All he's got is a fighting chance. You're his life line. I've watched you all these years. I guess I should have told you that before." He lifts his head and looks me in the eye. "You've been great."

"Thank you, Hal." I look straight back into his eyes. That is the only compliment I can take without flinching.

"I'll talk to the nurses. You do what you can for Peter."

"I hope I'm fighting on the right side."

"You are," he answers. "This time you are."

"I'm not sure, but I can't help it" is all I can say.

I'm making myself right at home here. I know my way around. I've got friends in high places. They know me in the coffee shop ("Half a teaspoon of sugar, no milk, right, hon?"). The woman behind the reception desk— once as welcoming as Cerberus—no longer requires that I stop for the requisite visitor's pass. I'm a regular. I belong.

"Good morning!" The receptionist smiles a greeting as I pass by, clutching Soft Gray to my breast, and a couple of magazines under my arm. Peter's orange Adidas T-shirt is flung over my shoulder. His arms look so thin poking out of the short sleeves, muscles wasted to fat, melting like tallow, collecting at his elbows. Still, it's his favorite shirt. Maybe it will cheer him up.

I move slowly and smoothly through the lobby of the new wing of the hospital to the brushed-steel elevators and push the call button. The "L" blinks pink as the elevator bounces onto the lobby and the doors float open.

Nobody dares to smile in the hospital elevator, except at newborn babies or to return a volunteer's smile. Volunteers smile for nothing. It is as if we knew that a casual smile might invade grief or worry, so we all hold our faces stiff and watch the numbers rise.

The door opens at 2. CORONARY reads the handsome, architect-designed bas-relief letters on the facing wall. A stubby-chic arrow points to the right. Enter a candy-striper, pert as Little Red Riding Hood in her pinafore, carrying a wire-basketful of clattering crimson test tubes. The doors close and I stare through the stenciled number 3, waiting for it to light up, waiting for the slow short drift to down, and the doors to open.

The new wing must end here. ICU is abbreviated for convenience in elongated block letters made of black electrical tape on the shabby wall. A tape arrow, fringed with stray torn strings, indicates left. The old white vinyl tile floors in the corridor gleam in overlapping circles and curlicues of waxy, reflected light. I know the routine. The grim reaper must have just passed through—a colored man, dressed in laundered, crumpled hospital blue, swinging his electric buffer before him like a scythe.

"Mary-Lou!" Dr. Braverman pops out from an intersecting corridor. "I was on my way out, but why don't I just walk you to ICU. We can talk on the way."

"Fine."

"What have you got there?" Dr. Braverman delicately removes the magazines from under my arm. *"Hot Rod* and *Hustler?"*

"I'm desperate," I explain. "I'll try anything."

"Well, it's working," says Dr. Braverman with a smile, tucking the magazines back under my arm. "I think you'd better carry them." We walk for a moment in silence.

"I was just looking at Peter's morning X-ray."

"How's the pneumonia?"

"Receding, but very slowly. That's what worries me. It would help our effort significantly if the pneumonia would clear up quickly. As things stand now, we're asking the impossible of him, and so far, he's delivering. This is day six and we've already got him down to 'half and half.' That's half machine breathing, half independent breathing. He might just make it. I have a feeling he will. When I assess his condition purely on the basis of the medical evidence—the X-rays, the blood gasses, the white-cell count—he shouldn't make it. But when I stop by to visit him, and I look at him, some sixth sense tells me he's going to. How are the nurses behaving?"

"At least they tolerate us now, you saw to that. Soft Gray's been invited back, grudgingly. I don't understand why they're so aloof, verging on nasty."

"You've got to understand, nurses and mothers are natural antagonists in an intensive care unit. They resent you, and you resent them."

"Granted. But there's more to it than that. That doesn't explain why them seem to resent Peter. How can they resent a kid who's fighting for his life? It's crazy. I see them fondle and coo at babies. I see them handle dying elderly people with such dignity and care even when they're comatose. It may be an act, but they perform it impeccably, and that's a kind of caring . . ."

"I don't understand it either. Perhaps it's partly your imagination."

"I don't think so. Actually, the only other time I saw them treat a patient more cruelly was two nights ago when they worked on a sixteen-year-old girl who had overdosed on drugs. They did a good job on her. She was out of ICU by the time I got in the next morning. But all the time they were working on her they seemed angry."

"It must be your imagination. They are an excellent team, the best."

"It's not a matter of competence. Anyhow, in spite of them, Peter seems to be getting better."

"How are you doing?"

We stop at the magic doors.

"Well. Remarkably well. I've gotten used to this place. I almost like it. I know that's weird, but you've got to be weird to survive here. I seem to be full of energy. I even managed to file my monthly column on time. A humor column, would you believe!"

"I'm beginning to believe anything. What's it about?"

"A much decorated schnook of a French soldier named Nicolas Chauvin, the guy who gave patriotism its bad name. I figure he's one of the unsung heroes of the women's liberation movement—after all, we're always invoking his name— so I thought I'd write about him."

"Who was the other unsung hero?"

"Some pig." I hit the square metal Stanley Magic Door button with my hip.

"Let me know if you need anything," Dr. Braverman calls over his shoulder, laughing, as the door arcs close, fanning his exit with a whoosh of air.

"Good morning," I say as I walk past the nurses' station on my way to Peter, but they do not return the greeting.

"G'morning, petunia puss. How are they hanging?" I glance up at the IV bags. Pete doesn't smile. I place Soft Gray by his side. "I brought Soft Gray back." But it's no go. "And your favorite shirt. Let's put it on." He shakes his head no. "How about *Hot Rod* magazine, or *Hustler*?" I dangle the bait before his eyes. He just stares.

I sit down by his bed and take his hand in mine, tubes and all, and kiss his fingertips where the tiny muscles are too atrophied to bend around the flannel-covered board on which hand and wrist are taped, to keep them motionless. The vein in his wrist is worn out. Now the intravenous antibiotic drips into the top of his hand.

"Look, Peter, I know that you're feeling discouraged. I know you're worried that you're not getting better, but you're wrong. It's going to be very tough, but you can do it if you want to. That's not just what *I* say. That's what Dr. Braverman thinks too.

"So far you're doing great. See?" I point toward the dial on the respirator. "It's set for six breaths per minute, assist control. Just yesterday it was set at twelve. That means that every minute you're breathing just as much as the machine. You're taking turns. That's great! That's a lot of progress for six days."

All the while I'm speaking, I am hearing my own voice. It sounds earnest and brave and MGM-innocent—like Judy Garland talking to Toto. That's a sure sign to me that I'm terrified. This is a very long way from Kansas. I hope, against all the evidence of reality, that Peter can't tell.

Peter blinks his eyes in rapid succession. I place the pen

between his fingers and reach for the clipboard. Holding the top with my left hand, I tilt the board at an angle, resting the bottom edge of the board on his belly. With my right hand I hold his arm up by lifting the wrist and supporting it delicately between the tips of my thumb and third finger. Instinctively I adjust my upward support so that it matches and thereby cancels out the downward pull of gravity.

He begins to write. Because I must be standing to support his moving hand properly, I cannot see what he is writing. His hand blocks my view.

I anticipate each frail stroke of each letter as if he were tracing with his finger on my bare back, the way when I was a girl we used to take turns at the beach, writing "I love you" on the lifeguard's back. We erased mistakes with our palms.

I stare at the top of his hand as it moves diagonally, from right to left, in a downward stroke. Then he lifts his hand up ever so slightly off the paper and makes another downward diagonal stroke—this one from left to right. I know it's going to be the letter *A* before he draws the final, horizontal line.

The next one is an *M*. He makes those strokes straight up and down, so I have to wait until the third stroke to make sure it's not an *N*.

I can't tell if the next one is going to be a *T* or an *I* or an *L* until he draws a horizontal line across the top and bottom, and then I know it's an *I*.

I'm pretty sure from the spherical way he starts out on the next letter that it's going to be an *O*, but I'm wrong. He stops in mid-circle and finishes it off as a *G*.

The next letter is an *O*. He is writing: *"AM I GOING TO DIE?"*

I wait until we're finished writing, until the dot is under the question mark, to answer him. I give myself that much time to think. Any more would be suspicious.

"No."

The white muslin curtain is drawn around patient number six, Mr. Wisznicki. Since he's in a coma, it doesn't much matter that he can't see out and the nurses can't see in. If he dies, bells will ring.

Beep, beep, beep, beep, beep. The incessant nag, nag, nag that a telephone makes when the circuits are busy assaults the air. It's Mr. Wisznicki's IV alarm. Time to hang another .05 dextrose and saline combo.

In unconscious response, the digits of Pete's cardiac readout flit back and forth with technological spriteliness, and then settle back to 123. Peter is asleep. I watch his chest rise and fall. The respirator is set for six breaths per minute, assist control. I can barely detect any movement in his chest when he breathes the eighteen breaths on his own. But every three breaths, when the respirator takes over, Pete's chest heaves high, and the machine sounds exasperated, like a teacher who has had to demonstrate something very, very simple too many times. It is the seventh day. One more to go. So far, so good.

A low gurgle, an almost human sound, like a descant, joins the nagging beep of the IV alarm. Mr. Wisznicki needs servicing.

Nurse C. Bocanfusco, her scissors swinging at her hip, scoots over from the central nurses' station on silent white rubber heels and whips the curtain open. The jolting zip of hundreds of little metal clips careening through metal track set in the ceiling sends Pete's digits flickering toward consciousness again.

"Shhhhhh!" I hiss in a stage whisper. "Pete's sleeping!" The bitch. She doesn't have to make that much noise. She could open the curtain gently.

She touches the red alarm light on the IV hook-up with her finger, and the beeping stops.

"I'm just going to detach your breathing tube for a second, Mr. Wisznicki," she calls loudly, a routine courtesy for the unconscious.

Mr. Wisznicki's eyes are shut. His toothless mouth would fall open in a collapsed little black "O" of a hole if it were not taped to form a seal around the respirator mouthpiece.

His whole face falls away from his nose, which like the over-large beak of a hungry baby bird points expectantly upward. I examine the skin on the huge bony hands, which are laid out, like exhibits, on top of the sheet. The flat blue veins seem to lie on top of the skin. The skin on his hands looks dry and scaly, as if it were made of pastry flakes. The respirator plays his chest like a bellows.

"I'm just going to empty out this condensation, all right?" Deftly, she twists off the flexible tube where it connects to the mouthpiece, spills out the water that has collected where the tube rests, bent against Mr. Wisznicki's chest, and reconnects the system without missing a beat. "Better?"

Mr. Wisznicki's vacant body answers with a lurch and a hiss. No more gurgle.

There are eight ages of man, not seven. Shakespeare didn't anticipate the miracles of modern medicine. It's the eighth one that's really "sans everything."

"While I'm here, Mr. Wisznicki, I'll change your sheets and freshen you up a bit with a little bed bath." Nurse C. Bocanfusco, her conversation on automatic pilot, looks up to draw the curtain closed. For a split second our eyes meet. "Now we'll just give ourselves a little privacy," she prattles on, closing the curtain with a noisy jerk. If it were a door, she'd slam it.

I go back to the business of watching Peter breathe. I place my hand across my chest, as if I were saluting the flag, and ration my breathing so that my breast rises no more than Peter's, so that I get no more air than he. I am about to panic and gulp air when the whoosh of Peter's respirator signals that I may take one regular breath. I can't believe that tomorrow he will be breathing on his own.

I reach for the clipboard at the foot of his bed and begin to read the various communications—some right side up, some upside down; some messy, some neat; some slanted, some overlapping; almost all incomplete—that cover the well-used sheet of paper like a collage of interrupted telegraph messages.

"*Scratch above my left . . .*" Somehow I knew he meant "ear." "*When's Daddy . . .*" He'll be here any minute. "*Bend my . . .*" Periodically Pete's knees get stiff, even though there's a pillow under them.

There are lots of large *X*'s scattered all over the page, the kind that could be kisses at the bottom of a letter, but they're not. They're shorthand for Xylocaine, as in "Throat hurts terribly."

We communicate so well that I can find only one completed message: "*Am I going to die?*" I press down on the clip with the heel of my hand, remove the page, crumple it and throw it into the basket. What was I supposed to answer: "Maybe"?

"Oh shit, oh shit, oh shit, shit, shit." A voice racked by sorrow and disbelief sounds from behind the curtain. It's not the Florence-Nightingale-out-of-Walt-Disney-robot voice of Nurse C. Bocanfusco, but it can't be Mr. Wisznicki. Something's wrong.

"What's the matter?" I pull aside the curtain. Nurse C. Bocanfusco is on her knees at Mr. Wisznicki's bedside.

"Are you all right?" I walk around the bed to help her up.

"I'm okay, thanks," she smiles wanly, getting herself up off the floor. "I'm fine, really. It's Mr. Wisznicki." She holds her hands up, offering them for inspection. "Stool."

"You mean shit."

"You're right." Nurse C. Bocanfusco starts laughing. "When you expect it, it's stool; when it surprises you, it's shit." She walks over to a nearby sink, nudges the lever located under the basin to "on" with her right knee and presses the flat of her left hand up and down against the metal nipple of the soap dispenser. "Does shit bother you, Mrs. Weisman?"

"Call me Mary-Lou. No, not at all. It's just about my favorite discharge."

"My name's Crystal." She holds out her hand.

"Mind if I don't?"

We both laugh while she rubs her palms downward on the

front of her skirt. "Well, back to work."

"Would you like me to help you with Mr. Wisznicki? I know how to make hospital corners."

"Thanks. I'd appreciate it."

She pulls the table that's been rolled down to the foot of the bed forward to about the level of Mr. Wisznicki's knees and places on it a large metal basin half-filled with water, a white washcloth, worn thin by industrial laundering, and a tiny rectangle of soap, the size you get in a hotel, complimentary. "Why don't you stand on the other side of the bed. I'll stay on this side," she instructs, dipping the washcloth in the basin. I step around the foot of the bed to the other side. "First we'll pull the sheet down. Gently. He has an in-dwelling catheter."

His penis surprises me. It lounges between his withered shanks, long, plump, pink and improbably robust. It's the only part of him that isn't old.

Crystal takes the washcloth from the basin and squeezes it slightly. "Reach over, grab on to his pelvis and roll him gently toward you. That's perfect. Hold him like that while I sponge his buttocks."

I watch her clean and rinse, clean and rinse. Silently, bendingly, like two Roman priestesses, we perform the ancient lustral rite of purification on the body of Mr. Wisznicki.

Mr. Wisznicki is much lighter than Pete. I've done this a lot of times with Pete, except that, since I'm usually alone, I hold his hip forward with my left hand, and then I reach around and wash his bottom with my right. Then, to do the other side, I have to move his bed away from the wall. That's not as difficult as it sounds. Hospital beds come on casters.

People in wheelchairs have a lot of trouble shitting, especially people in the late stages of muscular dystrophy when the involuntary muscles become, as they say, "involved." Peter takes Senakot. Sometimes when it doesn't work by morning the way it's supposed to, he has an accident at school and I have to go get him. That's bad enough.

It's even worse when the laxative doesn't work at all, and I have to help him by reaching up with my finger. We have a way of making it not nearly as humiliating as one might think. We call Senakot "semi-crap!" We call ourselves "asshole buddies." We say we're "teasing the turd."

Crystal drops the washcloth into the basin and places a clean towel on top of the soiled sheet. "Okay; you can let go now. I'll be back in a jiffy with some fresh water." I lower Mr. Wisznicki onto the towel.

Now it is my turn to wash; her turn to hold. I feel her eyes on me as I wash the inside of his thigh, his scrotum.

"Frankly, I had you figured all wrong." Crystal breaks the silence. "I thought you were one of those pain-in-the-ass mothers, Jewish princess variety. Most of them are. Even the ones who aren't Jewish."

"Frankly, I had you figured for a bitch. Why were you so mean to Peter, so mean to me? Why were you so angry about that girl?"

"What do you mean?" But I can tell Crystal knows what I mean. She lets out a long, heavy sigh. "Is it *that* obvious?" She lifts her head and looks at me. "Wow! I guess it is," she answers herself. "The truth is, I have to keep far enough away from death so I can fight it, far enough away so I can bear it when I lose. Here in ICU, you mostly lose. A young person, like the one we pumped out the other night, makes us furious. There she is in number eight, throwing her life away, while next door in seven, Pete is fighting for his."

"But that doesn't explain why—"

"No one threatens us more than Peter, more than you and Peter and your family with your terrifying, death-defying love. And it's not going to work. No matter how intensely you love him, or how well we care for him, he's going to die. I can't stand having to take care of kids who are going to die. I'm sorry. There's no excuse for the way I acted. I shouldn't be a nurse if I can't take it."

I let go of the washcloth for a moment to touch her hand. "Hey, sometimes I can't take being his mother. Yesterday

Pete asked me a question on his clipboard. He wanted to know if he was going to die. I think he meant was he going to die tomorrow, when Dr. Braverman takes him off the respirator. At least that's what I wanted him to mean, so that's how I interpreted it. In any event, I answered 'No.' I took the coward's way out. I've never told Peter that he's going to die."

"You may very well have interpreted his question correctly."

"But what if I haven't? What if he didn't mean tomorrow? What if he finally had found the courage to confront his own death, only to have me betray him by my cowardice? After all these years of him trusting me, I can't bear it if I've lied to him in the end."

"Then why not give him another chance to ask?" Crystal lowers Mr. Wisznicki's body and begins to pat him dry with a towel.

"How? How would I do that?"

"I'm not sure. I wouldn't do it now, in the hospital. I'd wait for the right time, a more pleasant time, when you are both feeling particularly close to each other and relaxed."

"But what should I say? How should I ask? I mean, I just can't say, 'Hey, by the way, Pete, a couple of weeks ago when you were in the hospital you asked me if you were going to die, and—' "

Crystal interrupts. "Of course you can't. When you find the right time, you'll find the right words. Trust your instincts. They've gotten you this far."

"Thanks. That sounds like good advice."

"Thank you for squaring with me. By the way—" Crystal reaches a wet hand into her pocket. "Here." She opens her palm and grins.

My very own vial of Xylocaine.

I am standing at the head of Peter's bed, holding his arms up and pulling them back over his head. "It will expand his chest and increase his lung capacity a little bit," Dr. Braver-

man has instructed. "That little bit might make a big difference. And anything else you can think of that might help,
anything that might serve to put him at ease. I'm going to
turn the respirator off completely, but I'm not going to tell
him. After two weeks on a respirator, he's bound to panic if I
announce when I'm turning it off. We'll wait a couple of
hours until we're confident he's going to make it on his own,
and then we'll tell him he's *been* off."

I have prepared Peter like a primitive warrior for battle.
Or an Egyptian for burial. The boisterous orange of his
Adidas T-shirt exaggerates the vulnerability of his em-
bryonic body. Like wet tissue paper, the skin of his upper
arms threatens to yield and break under the pressure of my
thumbs. Soft Gray, talisman and mascot, rests across his lap.
I've done my best, but the results seem naïve, as if there were
a God of kids to whom he is appealing.

The respirator hose is still attached to the plastic tube
protruding from Peter's mouth, even though the dials are
turned to zero. I lean over the head of his bed, waiting for his
next breath, my eyes fastened, as if mesmerized by a flickering flame, on the tentative rise and fall of his chest beneath
the orange shirt, waiting for a miracle. It is the eighth day.

"Do you know what day it is today?" I ask Pete, to keep
his mind off breathing. "July eleventh, 1979, the day Sky
Lab's supposed to fall to earth. Only, you don't have to
worry about getting hit in the head. It's falling in the Aus-
tralian desert. Might hit a kangaroo or two. That would
make them hopping mad, don't you think?"

I lean over farther to get a look at his face. The corners of
his mouth are slack around the tube. His eyes look dull and
dark.

"You know what kangaroos sing when they blow out their
birthday candles?" I race on with my words, like so many
colored triangular banners on a string trailing behind me.
"They sing 'Hoppy Birthday,' what else?"

Nothing. Not a glimmer. *Oh Jesus, help.*

"Dummmmm, dummmmm, dummmmm, da-a-ummmmmm!" It is the sound of a barbershop quartet tuning up in ascending thirds, and ending with a final, syncopated flourish. It is Adam and Larry, their heads peering around the sides of the curtain like two hand puppets. They step into the cubicle and belt out a brazen "Ta-daa" against the gloom.

"Hey, Pete! Look at Daddy. Look at Addie. Aren't they funny?" I hate how desperate I sound.

"I brought you the July issue of *Penthouse,* buddy boy. Terrific headlights, and you should see what else . . ." Adam opens the magazine to the centerfold and holds it in front of Pete's face. "Split beaver!"

"For Chrissakes, guys," I protest, "that's gross, really gross. I don't ever want to hear you say that again."

Peter loves it when I scold like a parody of a mother. He loves it when I flail around the kitchen, falling on my knees, beseeching God to give me strength. But not this time. I think I see light in those depleted eyes for a second, but maybe not.

"Guess what we ate for breakfast?" says Larry, ignoring Pete's indifference. "Go ahead, guess."

Larry reaches for the clipboard. "Let go of his arms for a minute, M'Lou, Pete's got to write." He places the pen in Peter's limp fingers and holds them over the clipboard. "Go ahead, guess." Pete drops the pen, on purpose.

"All right, then, you lazy slob, I'll tell you. Beans. We had beans. Didn't we?" Adam nods vigorously.

"Prove it?" says Larry. "Is that what you're thinking, 'prove it'? He doesn't believe me," Larry complains in a mocking tone. "He wants me to prove it. Shall I?"

"Yes," we intone eagerly.

"Okay," says Larry. Looking very serious, he sticks out his pointer finger at Peter. He reaches for Pete's right hand and lifts it from where it rests on the sheet. "Pull my finger, Petie. Not too hard, though. Go ahead; pull my finger."

We watch Peter's thin, bony fingers creep around Larry's and effect a tiny tug.

The intensive care unit rings with the sound of farts, a veritable opera of farts, a lower intestinal extravaganza, a virtuoso performance.

A rich baritone recitative gives way to staccato coloratura yips, as if our heroine were fleeing danger. Then, without warning, the timbre drops to basso profundo for a few Gregorian blasts before it spikes again to a hair-raising countertenor. Larry's eyes bulge. The tendons stand out in his neck. Pausing to take a breath, he descends the register, *glissando,* to tenor range, piercing the room with the melody of romantic hyperbole. Just when it seems there can be no more, not possibly, he presses his hands together like a diva, and squeezes one last heroic little quack of a grace note past his weary sphincter.

Peter is laughing. I can tell by the smile around the tube, the drool spilling onto his chain, the twinkle in his eyes and the rapid, rabbity dilation of the wings of his nostrils. Under the sheets, I can see that he is rubbing his legs together in an excess of delight, like a weak cricket.

Adam and I double over and step around the bed, heel-toe, like Indian dancers, alternately holding our hands to our mouths to muffle the escaping hilarity, and slapping our hands on our thighs in some lordy-lordy reflex of mirth.

Larry presides over all with a proud grin.

"What's going on in here?" Crystal pokes her head through the curtain. I wish I could stop laughing and tell her, but I can't. There is nothing so funny as a fart. It is humor itself, the body's own pratfall, an unsolicited comment on the human condition. The fart is the original pie in the face, the inaugural punch line.

"What's that funny smell?" Crystal screws up her face into a quizzical, frustrated little clench, as if the answer were just approaching the outskirts of her olfactory zone.

With a conditioned response as old as grammar school, I raise an accusing finger, point to the cubicle next door and manage to whisper discreetly through the giggles and gasps,

"I think it's coming from Mr. Wisznicki."

"Oh," says Crystal with an understanding smile, "I'd better go check. I'll see you guys later," she adds, pulling the curtain closed.

"Now, Mr. Wisznicki," we hear her yelling courteously in the first-person plural comatose impersonal, "we're just going to roll you over on your side and have a look . . ."

I glance at Peter. His chest flutters tympanically with laughter and breath. His eyes gleam. His cheeks glow.

He has done it. He is going to be all right. For this one, last time, everything is going to be all right.

It crosses my mind as we stand around Peter's bed smiling, that we are learning to be very grateful for very little, and I wonder for a fleeting moment if we are pitiful.

"There's Spellman!" Peter stage-whispers from his place at the end of the kitchen table, from which he has the best view of the new Audubon bird feeder. It's supposed to be squirrelproof, but it's not, at least not to the arch villain of our bird-watching dramas, Wally Wallenda.

Standing at the kitchen window in my bathrobe, looking through the mist rising off my morning coffee, I can see Wally crouched on the limb of a nearby tree, getting up his nerve, waiting for his command. If it's "go," his gray, furry body will coil and then hurl itself through the air, back legs stretched, front paws reaching, claws curling, anticipating their grip on the feeder's edge.

"And there's *Mrs.* Spellman!" says Pete, as a second cardinal, its glory beautifully muted by buff, perches on the feeder's edge, light as flame, quick as spirit. Wally Wallenda waits.

We watch the birds hunt and peck, their tiny heads staccato and humorous with intent. Wally pounces. His nails skid off the feeder's plastic dome. Foiled again. He drops through the air humiliated and graceless, scrambling for a landing. In a red frenzy of flutter, the cardinals abandon the feeder and disappear into the azalea bushes.

"Shhh!" says Peter, as if that would bring them back. But it's too late.

I stand at the kitchen window, staring out over my cup, mesmerized by and yet not quite focused on the bird feeder swaying gently from a wire stretched between two trees.

I wonder how much he knows. "Everything, everything," my friends all agree. "He's *got* to know by now. He's got to have heard it, or figured it out by now."

But I'm not so sure. I, who probably know him best and most; I'm not so sure. And if he knows, how much does he know? Does he know how soon? Does he want to know?

And if he has this dreadful knowledge, and I don't know it, does that mean he does not want to share it with me, which is okay, I guess, if it's a choice, but what if it means he is too terrified to speak of it, and perhaps not just to me, but to his own consciousness? What if he lives isolated in dread and torment? That might be crueler, even, than the knowledge of death. Instinct tells me this is the right time.

"Pete?"

"What, Mom."

"Pete . . . If you had to go back to the hospital . . . if you, you know, caught another cold like the last one—"

"You know I don't like to talk about those things," Pete interrupts.

"Okay, then, we won't. I just want you to know that if you ever change your mind, I'm not too scared to talk about it."

"Mom . . . ?"

"What, Pockie."

"Scratch behind my left ear."

I scratch.

"A little higher, and more to the left."

I scratch a little higher, and more to the left.

"Thanks, you got it. Now, pick up my right hand, please. I've got a crumbly in the corner of my eye."

Together we defy gravity. I take his elbow with one hand and his wrist with the other, and guide them upward until his hand hangs slack in front of his eye. There is still a tiny pastel smudge of blue and yellow on the top of his right hand where the intravenous needle was inserted.

He moves his head so that his waiting thumb makes light contact with the eyelid, like a phonograph needle set gently down upon a record. Then he moves his head from side to side, rubbing the corner of his eye back and forth against his static thumb.

"Thanks," he says, inspecting his thumb with a Jack Hornerish smile. "I got it. Now I want to eat breakfast. Put my right elbow inside, between my side and the arm of my wheelchair. Put the spoon in my hand. Lift up my left hand and put it on the table . . . No," he corrects me patiently, "I don't want to hold the bowl, I just need my left arm propped out there for balance. Move the cereal bowl more to the upper right. Okay. That's good . . . Nope, I spoke too soon," he says, musing over the distance from hand to bowl, and concludes that the present angle at which his right arm is cocked will not allow the spoon to reach all the way to the cereal, never mind all the way back to his mouth. "Make my right arm a little longer. Pull it up. Just a bit. A teensy bit. Less than an inch, but no more than a milli-mousefart." A milli-mousefart is Peter's idea of the smallest measurable unit of force.

We are mad inventors. Together we make Rube Goldberg machines out of the unused parts of his body. His torso and right and left arms make a tripod at the kitchen table for his head. This time we are going to make a feeding machine. It works on Archimedes' theory of the lever. The machine is activated when the head drops to the side, over the left shoulder. Acting as a counterweight, the head pulls the upper torso slightly to the left.

The oblique angle of the leftward leaning torso acts like a lever, exerting upward pressure on the right elbow, which is held in place, tucked between the rib cage and the inside of the wheelchair arm rest. That upward pressure counteracts the normal downward pull of gravity, thereby allowing the lower arm to swing to and fro freely on the fulcrum of the elbow, resulting in the delivery of food to the mouth.

The spoon, so carefully balanced, slips away from Peter's limp fingers and clatters onto the floor.

"Crash-tinkle, it fell to the floor," Peter sings. "Crash-tinkle" is the euphemism for books that slide off his lap, or milk that spills at him, creeping across the table, curling off the edge, and for all the other indignities that he is helpless to stop.

I put the spoon back into his limp-wristed hand, lace his fingers around the handle and squeeze them into a grip. Just give me a place to stand, I pray with Archimedes, and I can move the world. But the fingers loosen slowly, as soon as I let go, and the spoon falls.

"Maybe we ought to reconsider ordering those ball-bearing feeders that Dr. Tierney showed us."

Ball-bearing feeders are prosthetic metal devices, shiny steel tendons and bones, which mimic the arm's natural machinery. They look as if they belong in a dentist's office, eerily holding up the drill, or wherever radioactive material is handled. Their purpose is to offset the downward pull of gravity, thereby enhancing the power and range of the weakened person's every move. Ball-bearing feeders are the next best thing to living on the moon.

The "shoulders" are just metal brackets which must be fastened tightly about halfway up each of the frame's vertical metal tubing to which the vinyl back rest is riveted. From these "shoulders" hang the "upper arms," two metal rods and a sinewy metal cable. The wheelchair's armrests have to be removed in order to accommodate the well-oiled elbows and the long narrow metal troughs into which the patient's lower arms rest. The hands hang limp from the ends of the metal troughs as from a sling. Calibrations are made at the elbows with a special little wrench, according to just how much strength and range the patient has. Peter has hardly any. When he writes a paper for school, or a letter, he prints faintly and in an area the size of a newspaper column.

"You'd be able to feed yourself more smoothly"—I mean "better," but I say "more smoothly"—"and you'd be able to use more of the paper when you write and draw."

"I'm enough of a machine already," Pete says.

My eyes take in his sad inventory: the polyurethane wings that hold him up under his arms as if he were perpetually being dragged, headfirst, boot heels scraping in the dust, out of a saloon in a cowboy movie, and the joy stick, the drive box, the motors, the seat belt, the drive belts, the batteries, the cables, the wires, the wheels.

Pete looks me cold in the eye. "No more. I'd rather be dead."

I pick up his spoon.

"Feed me like a mommy bird," says Pete, and we invent the mommy-bird feeding machine.

I set the spoon back down on the table and make a big deal out of picking it up with my teeth, which makes Pete laugh. Holding the handle of the spoon in my mouth like a crane, I manage to scoop up a little cereal. I move my head forward toward his wide-open mouth.

"Tweet!" Petie pipes, grinning at me conspiratorially. "Tweet! I'm a baby bird." Not a helpless child; a baby bird.

Laughing, I let the spoon fall from my mouth onto the table.

"Crash-tinkle!" Peter laughs back.

"Oh, Pockety-Pock!" I can't stop covering his face with kisses. "I love you. You're the best kid in the whole world."

"You're really very fortunate to have a kid like me," Peter agrees. "You could have had a real spoiled brat."

"You're absolutely right. That would have been awful."

"But, of course, if you hadn't been lucky enough to have me, and you had a brat instead, you probably wouldn't feel too bad about it because you wouldn't know me, anyway, so you wouldn't know what you were missing."

"That's true," I say, kissing the tip of his nose, "but I still count my blessings that I have a child as wonderful as you."

"I wouldn't count my blessings if I were you," says Pete.

"You wouldn't? Why not?"

"Because it sounds too pathetic."

I know before Peter says, "There's something sticky on my leg," what it is. The smell of his sperm, mushroomy and rank with mock fecundity, assails my nostrils.

"Let's see," I say as lightly as I can, pulling the sheet down tentatively, as if I had been called upon to identify a mutilated body in a morgue. His penis rests in a tangled triangle of dark hair between thighs as silky and white and plump with fat as a woman's. The smell of a man rises from his crotch.

"I think you've had a wet dream!" I announce, as if it were his first tooth, his first step or his first word instead of macabre life signs, like fingernails still growing on a dead man, or an erection at a hanging. Biology is a fanatic that knows no mercy. I will be brazen too. "Congratulations!"

"Congratulations for what? It feels bad; it smells bad. Yuck!" He wiggles his nose. "I hate it. Please wash it off me."

"Congratulations on becoming a man. That's terrific."

"I don't see anything so terrific about it."

"What's so terrific about it, for one thing . . ." I stall for courage, turning on the faucets in his bathroom, holding a basin under the nozzle, waiting for the water to run warm. "For one thing, it means you can have sexual intercourse."

"You mean fucking?" Peter calls back.

"Precisely."

I return to his room and set the basin on the bureau. To keep the mattress dry, I push a towel with my fingertips beneath his buttocks and upper thighs, as if it were a diaper. I reach into the basin for the washcloth. The warm water laps against my wrists. The soap nuzzles my hand. I wring out the cloth and begin to scrub. The sweet pastel scent from the soap makes the room as fragrant as a nursery.

"Ooooooooh, we'll scrub him and we'll flub him and we'll dub him in the derrière, we'll send him with a pigeon or whatever is a carr-i-ere . . ." I improvise a Gilbert and Sullivan patter song as I dip the cloth in and out of the basin, scrubbing gently at the crusty deposits on his inner thighs. "We'll clean him up and powder him and make him so de-lish-e-ous, that you will never know that once he smelled just like a fish-e-ous." Pete chortles with glee. I bend over and kiss him, and for that brief, stolen moment I know that what my desperate biology wants is to take my manchild-baby back, to swallow him down, deep and safe and forever inside me.

"There," I conclude, kissing his bellybutton. "You're divine. Now let's get you dressed for school. We'll have to hurry or you'll be late." I open his bureau and toss out a pair of underpants, some socks and his favorite green turtleneck shirt and green trousers. "How about going as a string bean today, okay?"

"Okay."

"It's really cold this morning. Fall is definitely over. Maybe you'd better wear a sweater under your ski jacket."

"I can't bend my arms when I'm wearing so many layers," Pete complains. "I can hardly drive wheelie."

"I know, pumpkin puss, but it's important that you be warm."

Automatically now, my mind translates the bitter, black truth into palatable white lies, half-truths and distortions. What am I supposed to say—"Bundle up, Peterkins, or you'll catch your death of cold"?

"I'd rather be dead than have to wear all those clothes," says Peter, and I wonder if he speaks the idiom or the truth. We play a dangerous game these days, devilishly near the brink.

There is no answer, so I gather up the left pants leg into a fat hoop of fabric, loop it around his left foot and begin to pull it up the leg. One of us will have to change the subject.

"Mom? How can I fuck?"

I know that what he really means is, "How can I fuck if I can't move?"

"That just shows how much you know about fucking! I

suppose the only way you know about is when the man lies on top of the woman and moves his penis in and out of her, right?"

Pete nods his head solemnly, shyly, although a soupçon of a smile titillates the corners of his mouth, anticipating with perfect faith from my strident tone that I have the answer.

With both feet in the leg holes, I grab the elastic waistband and pull upward, first tugging at the left side, then at the right, until the pants are on. A final tug at each cuff smooths out the wrinkles. "Well, you little male chauvinist piglet, did it ever occur to you that the man could lie on the bottom and the woman could lie on top and do all the moving?"

"Does that work, or are you just making it up?" Peter asks, the smile taking over as if it were spilled on his face.

"It works all the time," I grin back. "Lots of people prefer sex that way. Even people who aren't handicapped."

"Really?" His smile dazzles.

"Really."

"Who do I fuck? When do I start?"

Trying to imagine who, I pull the turtleneck over his head, stretching the front out so it won't feel too tight slipping down over his nose and mouth, and feed his right hand through the sleeve, like a safety pin towing a broken elastic. I know. A surrogate. A nice person, young and understanding; pretty, too. What the hell. Why shouldn't she be pretty? I'll arrange for her to meet Pete in some natural way so he won't suspect—maybe at a rock concert. Adam will take him; that way it'll be even better. First they'll get to be friends, just like anybody else. I'll tell her not to rush it, to make it happen like a romance. And then . . . But I know that's never going to happen. I don't have to worry about that.

"Hang on! Hold your horses!" I tease. "You're still a bit too young. Just because you *can* do it doesn't mean you *have* to do it."

"I don't get it," says Peter, clearly disappointed. "What's the good of having wet dreams if I can't fuck yet?"

"Well, I've never had one, of course, but I always heard that the dreams are very exciting," I say, folding his left arm closed so that the hand can fit into the armhole.

"That's what I thought too," says Pete. "But it's not fair. I was gypped. I didn't have the dream. I just had the wet."

"Cunt, pussy, gash, snatch, fuzzy, cunt . . ." Peter recites.

"You already said 'cunt,' " says Adam. "You left out vagina, you doofus. How'd I ever get such an asshole for a brother!"

"And to think we walked out of an X-rated movie and into this!" Larry whispers in my ear. Still in our overcoats, the snow from our boots puddling the hall floor, we are scrunched down in front of the keyhole to Adam's room. The coital bump and grind of rock music emanating from the room, tuned to several notches above the parental noise-pollution standards, masks our whispering. The maniacal singer, twanging away at his electric guitar, hollers through cocaine-corroded vocal cords, as musical as the sound of a subway heard through a sewer grating. There is really no need to whisper.

"I've always wanted to know what they did when we went out on Saturday nights."

"We really shouldn't be doing this," Larry says. But he doesn't mean it. He always says the right thing first, just to get it out of the way. I always call his bluff.

"Maybe you're right. This is an invasion of their privacy. We'd better go. We'll just tiptoe out of the house and go get a cup of coffee or something, and then come back at the expected time." I often overdo it.

"Shut up, we're staying."

We settle in against each other, shoulder to shoulder, balancing precariously on the soles of our boots.

I love to spy. My body is rigid with excitement. A place on the front of my ankle where the folds of my boot are digging in hurts, but the pain is part of the fun. Peter in his wheelchair is in clear view.

When I first set eyes upon him, even after I have been away for just a little while, is when I really see him. His head is so large. His soft cheeks have begun to droop, as in middle age. His arms are thin and oddly shaped, like the white, stuffed arms of old-fashioned rag dolls. They are carefully angled on his armrests so they won't fall down and waggle, as if they hardly belonged to him. His lower legs hang, bowed with disuse. His stocking feet are arched like the backs of dolphins, the toes pointing straight down to the floor. His huge chest collapses like a sack full of grain, spreading his waistline wide. But there is a big smile on his face.

"How about all the words for masturbate?" A disembodied, callow male voice calls out over the music. It sounds like Adam's friend Yeager. Yeager collects Krugerrands. His father is a stockbroker.

"Well," says Peter with a shy smile, "I don't know any."

"Then we'll have to teach you. These are important things to know." Yeager moves into view and sits down on the floor in front of Pete, his back to us. "Want another piece of pizza?"

"I've already had three," says Pete.

"So what?" Yeager says grandiosely. "Your mom's not here. Have four. We're all having four, aren't we, guys? Open up, Weisman!"

"There's 'twanging the wire,' " says Adam, "and 'beating your meat'—"

"Or 'beating your pud,' " Yeager interrupts.

"Should we count that as one or two?" Adam asks.

"Let's count it as two," says Yeager, getting up and moving out of view.

Now I can see that Peter is laughing out of control. His nostrils are rabbity; he gasps for air. He can no longer breathe enough to laugh. "I like 'twanging the wire' best. That's what I'm going to call it," he says when he can speak. "Would one of you assholes please wipe my face? The tomato sauce burns my lips." A forearm appears in front of Pete's face and wipes his mouth on its sleeve.

"What about 'jerking off'?" O'Malley lumbers into view, indignant. O'Malley is large and dough-white Irish. He stuffs a Mallomar into his mouth, feeding the mixture of baby fat and muscle that upholsters his ungainly frame like mashed potatoes flung at an armature. O'Malley is trying to keep his weight up for football.

"You're gay, O'Malley," says Yeager for no particular reason.

"Take a chill pill," says Adam.

"Yeah, O'Malley, take a chill pill," Peter repeats, very rough, very tough, very cool. A white paper plate with a crust of pizza on it rests precariously on his sloping lap.

"Hey," says Adam, taking a place on the rug in front of Peter, "I forgot to tell you guys about a weird thing that happened at the gym today." Bare-chested, he wears a blue bandanna around his neck, and faded navy-blue sweat pants. His body is flawless and well-muscled. He works out at a gym. He drinks protein. When I talk to him, he gazes at his own reflection in my belt buckle. Crouched down, his back facing me, his elbows resting on his knees, I can see what he means about the importance of having well-developed *latissimi dorsi*. "I was working out on the lat machine and this fag—his name is Owen, I think he's in your home-room, Yeager . . ."

"O-wen, oh, O-wen!" Peter sing-songs girlishly, making a weak little flapping movement, a homosexual parody, with his wrist. "You dropped your purse!"

The room rings with the sound of adolescent braying. Peter beams with pleasure.

"Anyhow," Adam continues, "Owen came over to me and said, 'Was that your mother and brother I saw you with downtown in Friendly's last Saturday?' I was gonna tell him to fuck off, but I figured what the hell, so I said, 'Yeah.' And then Owen said, 'Why is your brother in a wheelchair?' "

Emergency! Emergency! The neural alarm is sounding in my brain, as once again I feel those words searing, branding deep into my chest.

"And what did you say to him, Adam? What did you say?" Peter asks, grinning with happiness, confident that because the story is from Adam, it has a happy ending.

"Well, I tried to figure out what you would have said to him if you'd been there, so I answered, 'Because he can't walk.' "

Pete smiles as if to say, "You did just right."

"So then," says Adam, "he asked me seriously what was wrong with you."

Wrong with you. The pain burns deeper and wider in my chest. Words will ever harm me.

"And so I told him that you had muscular dystrophy. And then he said, 'Gee, I'm sorry. That's real bad.' And then I said"—and here Adam's voice crescendos triumphantly—" 'Not as bad as being a fag'!"

Peter blushes with delight while the other guys hee-haw and slap their worn denim knees.

"How soon before your parents get home?" O'Malley sobers up. "I mean, do we have time for a brew?"

"Notice"—Larry nudges me with his shoulder—"they don't even call it beer."

"Sure," says Adam, glancing at his watch. "The movie gets out at eleven." I see Adam reach behind the sign I bought him at Parsell's Garden Mart last spring—KEEP OFF GRASS—that he keeps at the back of his desk, leaning against the corkboard wall, and produces a can of Miller's and a straw.

"Miller's is shit," says O'Malley.

"Then eat shit," says Adam, and they all bray some more.

"Go ahead, Pete, you go first," says Yeager, punching the top and slipping the straw into the can.

"What about Mom?" Peter glances at Adam.

"Fuck Mom. What she doesn't know can't hurt her. You're not going to tell her, are you? Promise?" Adam sounds a little panicky. Peter has trouble keeping secrets.

"No way," says Pete, taking a suck from the straw. "Good brew," he pronounces. "I like it."

"Good man," says O'Malley.

"It's time for you to go to bed, buddy boy. Mom and Dad are going to be home soon, and we don't want them to catch us. Otherwise, we won't be able to do this again next Saturday night."

"But you haven't shaved me yet. You said you were going to shave me!"

"We'll do it next Saturday night. I think your beard will hold until then," says O'Malley. I see him stroke upward on Peter's cheek with the back of his big, rough hand. "Just barely," he adds. "Pretty soon you're going to have to start shaving once a week. It's a bitch."

"Maybe I'll grow a beard," says Pete.

"You'd look cool with a beard," Yeager allows.

"Well, now you know what they do when we go out Saturday nights," says Larry, helping me to stand up. My feet are pins and needles. I fall against him. When his face grazes mine, it rubs away a tear I don't know about.

"Why are you crying?" he whispers, touching my face with his glove.

"I don't know," I sniff, smiling up at him because I really am fine. "I guess it's just this whole scene ... It's so, so ... normal."

"Will you be wanting the room for just the one night, sir?" The lady behind the desk at the Westport New Englander Motel eyes me suspiciously, or at least it seems that way to me. If she only knew. I fold my arms across my chest, making a point of exposing my wedding ring before I realize that the joke's on me. I could have bought it in a dime store.

"Actually, we'll only be needing it for a couple of hours," Larry answers rakishly.

"In that case we can give you our reduced rate," she replies, very businesslike. "That'll be eleven dollars, payable in advance. Do you have any luggage?" She sees damn well that we don't.

"No." Larry seems to be enjoying every minute of this. I wonder how he has signed the register. Probably "Mr. and Mrs. Smith."

"By the way," he says, making matters worse, "would you please give us a room with a bed that has magic fingers?"

"All our beds are equipped with magic fingers," she replies as if it were a source of pride.

"Good. Here's twelve dollars. I'd like four quarters for the extra dollar. The bed takes quarters, doesn't it?"

"One quarter will give you ten minutes of magic fingers," she says, sliding the quarters, along with the key, across the counter top. "It's the last door on the right at the end of the hall, number ten."

"By the way," Larry says, pausing to drop the quarters into his trouser pocket. They make a big racket landing. "We've given the motel's phone number to our kids, in case they need us. If one of them should call, please put the call through to the room."

"Now she's really bewildered," I giggle as Larry steers me down the carpeting. "This is crazy. Maybe we should just go to the movies."

"These are desperate times," says Larry, fitting the key into the lock and giving it a turn, "requiring desperate measures."

"I don't know if I can do it," I confess. "I don't know if I can relax enough. I'm a wreck."

"I know," he says, beginning to unbutton my blouse. "Don't worry about that. I'll relax you." He pulls my arms out of the blouse as if I were a child. "You're beautiful." He undoes the metal snap at the top of my jeans, releases the zipper and draws them slowly, along with my underpants, over my hips and down to my knees. "Beautiful," he whispers, kissing my navel. His dark curls are flecked with gray.

I look down at my belly. I can see where the waistband has furrowed my skin, where the round grommet has indented my skin; even where the zipper has left its mark. "I am getting old. My stomach looks like a topographical map of the land of Levi," I complain before I wish I hadn't.

But he does not protest at my protest. "So am I" is all he says, unlacing my sneakers.

Hobbled by my dungarees, my bare skin contracting into a chill, gray armoring, I stand rigid, begging myself to relax.

"What you need is a warm bath. You shouldn't be wearing sneakers in January." He takes them off, places them near the baseboard heating and walks to the bathroom. I step out of my dungarees, shaking them loose until they slide over my bare feet and onto the floor. *Wadami, wadami, wadami gonna do,* my brain churns as I stand frigid, untouchable, unyielding.

The sound of running water fills my head with its soft tumult of white music. Oh dear God, I want to feel. Please let me feel.

"Come here, darling."

Obediently I move across the floor. He kneels at the tub, his shirt sleeves rolled, a tiny pink bar of soap in one hand, a washcloth in the other. "Get in."

I break the surface with my toes. The water folds around my foot, warm, enveloping. The other foot follows. My palms pressed against the cold white sides of the tub, I lower my body ceremoniously, feeling each millimeter of the sweet torture as my body hardens and grows soft, and I sink into my element.

"Nice." I extend my legs in front of me, until my toes touch, and let my head fall back slowly, dipping my hair, feeling it float, touching me on the shoulder, reminding me of how good.

"Good," I murmur, feeling the word sound low, long and luxurious in my outstretched throat. "Good."

The water insinuates against my scalp, tickling among the hairs, closing about my head like fingers, drawing me in, as if I were being unborn. "Heaven."

The washcloth in Larry's hand glides over my body, nuzzling here and there like a cat's tongue. "Shoo-shoo, baby, shoo-shoo," he croons as the water laps enticingly at the hollows of my ears. "Shoo-shoo, baby, shoo-shoo." He lifts my foot from the water, cradling my heel in his hand. He kisses each toe before he pokes the tip of the washcloth between them and draws its roughness smoothly through the secret furrows.

After he soaps each breast slowly, following its roundness to the cold-crumpled nipples, I ease my torso beneath the water's surface and watch the bubbles drift away and dissipate and my breasts bloom pink. "Shoo-shoo, baby, shoo-shoo." His hand supports the nape of my neck, inviting me to surrender my weight. He touches my brow like a benediction. I close my eyes. I feel his fingertips comb through my hair, floatingly against my scalp, as if he would soothe my soul. I give myself over to the authority of his love.

"Better?" he whispers after a while.

"Much better." I reach my arms up, clasp my hands, wet and warm, around the back of his neck, and draw his face down to mine. "I love you, Larry." His lips soften and grow moist against mine. "I love the way you take care of me."

"I love taking care of you."

"Uh-oh. I've got an awful feeling . . ." I turn his wrist to read his watch. "It's almost eleven. We'd better go home and relieve Adam." I climb out of the tub, an aura of warmth clinging like memory to my skin.

"There's so little time for us," says Larry.

"There will be soon enough."

"We didn't even have time to make love." Larry wraps a towel around my shoulders.

"Yes we did." I slide my hands under his arms and press my damp face to his chest. I can feel the silky mat of hair beneath his shirt. "Yes we did."

"But what about the magic fingers?" He smiles, reaching into his trouser pocket and jangling the quarters.

"The magic fingers were terrific, too."

* * *

The back wheels of Peter's chair churn through the new-fallen snow, flinging out behind them little dots and dashes of powder compacted in the treads, which fall back down, nearly obliterating his tracks. "Is it good packing snow?"

I stop pushing the wheelie, reach down and scoop up a handful of snow, pat it together into a ball and lob it playfully onto Peter's lap. "What do you think?"

"Pretty good." He speaks softly and smiles as if he is imagining a snowball fight. "Let's take a real long walk. Besides, it's almost dinnertime." He stops to catch his breath every two or three words.

"Okay. But you're sure you're not too cold?" My breath steams like a dragon's before my face.

"I'm sure," says Pete. His words leave not a trace.

We walk in silence for a while, down the deserted street, watching the snow overwhelm and unite the angular pieces of our neighborhood, the roof lines and the roadways, into one swell of whiteness.

"Mom . . . ?"

"What, Pete."

"Did you know that in the olden times, Westport had lots of onion farms?"

"Really?"

"Mr. Sherwood, a relative of one of the early settlers, talked to our social studies class today. He told us about when Westport was a busy trading port. We shipped cargoes of onions to New York and sailed to the West Indies for rum."

"Really? I never knew that."

Pete grins, thrilled to be telling me something I do not know. "Yup! And you know what else he said? He said that everything we have on land—the trees, the rocks, the plants, the animals—everything is duplicated in the sea. He said there were mountains as tall as the Rockides and fish that looked like geese!"

"And what do you think?"

"I think that's probably mostly bullshit. I have a feeling

he had maybe imported a little too much rum." Peter smiles his special smile at me, sly and worldly-wise, yet a bit tentative in its cynicism, as if he is reluctant to abandon innocence and wonder altogether.

"I think maybe you're right."

"Anyway, he was a lot more interesting than the fire chief. All *he* did was talk about looking for frayed wires and how not to play with matches. What does he think we *are,* little kids?" Pete pauses for a moment of rhetorical indignation. "I'm not sure I believe in Santa Claus anymore," Peter goes on, "because if there really is a Santa Claus, don't you think it's kind of suspicious that Margaret Mead or somebody like her hasn't found him by now?"

I laugh out loud.

"Mr. Sherwood said that some of the sailors who sailed to the West Indies didn't know how to swim."

"Really? Doesn't that seem kind of dumb and dangerous for people who spend so much of their lives at sea?"

"That's what I thought too, but Mr. Sherwood said that they don't want to know how to swim. That way, if they get shipwrecked, they just drown."

"Don't they want to be saved?"

"Sure. But if there's no one around to rescue them, they figure they're better off not knowing how to swim. It would just prolong their agony."

"Oh."

"Mr. Sherwood said that even today lots of sailors and fishermen don't know how to swim. He said lots of times the Coast Guard finds life jackets floating with no men in them. They wear the life jackets for a while, but when the water gets too cold for them, and they know they're going to die before they're rescued, they take off the jackets and let themselves drown. See that tree over there?" Pete changes the subject with the easy abruptness of a small child with a short attention span and no agenda. He gestures with his head. "See how the trunk curves on the way up? It's a handicapped tree; it's got scoliosis, just like me."

"It's a wonderful, lovable, handicapped tree." My heart fills with homesick joy for the bittersweet harvest of his mind.

"Look, Mommy, look up. The clouds are darker than the night around them," Pete observes, allowing his heavy head to roll backward, baring his white warm neck to the cold light of the moon. "I don't think I ever saw the sky look that way before. It's like day and night are inside out. And if you look even deeper, you can see that the universe really is like a ball, a big round ball. Look, Mommy, look up. See? You can't get into it, and you can't get out of it, and you can be right side up, and upside down at the same time!"

I let my head fall back. Snowflakes land on my face and are warm and wet and gone in an instant, like tiny kisses. "It's true. It doesn't begin or end."

"And see how cold the trees are. The branches are gray and stiff with cold, like witches' fingers, but if you look at them real hard, with magic staring eyes, you can see that they have spring inside them. You almost have to imagine the green, but it's there if you can see it."

And, for a moment, in the twinkling of an eye, everything makes a kind of sense to me, beyond the ability of my eyes to see, or my reason to understand. The universal perspective, benign and anonymous, comforts me. "You know, Pete?" I feel my words tug at my throat, stretching the skin taut. "The universe is really a very well-ordered place, perfectly designed, everything in its proper place, playing its proper role. It's really all perfect, don't you think?"

"Just so long as you don't take it personally," says Peter. "Pick my head up, please."

We stop in our tracks. I turn and reach my mittened hand behind the nape of his neck and lift his head upright, until I sense that perfect, perilous point of equipoise.

Over Pete's shoulder I see a dark figure rushing toward us through the snow. I tuck the afghan under his legs and pull his wool cap farther down until his ear lobes disappear. I remove his hand from the joy stick and bring his cold fingers to my mouth to blow on them. This year I have had to cut the fingers off of his right glove so he can drive, so tenuous is his grip.

"Let's turn around and head for home. Daddy must have dinner ready by now."

"What are we having?"

"Macaroni and cheese."

"I hope it doesn't taste like soap."

"Do you think macaroni and cheese tastes like soap?" I pay attention to my tongue, trying to cross-match the sensations of soap with macaroni and cheese.

"Sometimes. And sometimes it tastes like candles."

"Wait up! Wait up!" It is a woman, dressed in a black coat, black galoshes flapping, arms waving, breath steaming. As she approaches, I feel an indeterminate dread.

I have never seen this woman before, and yet she is familiar—the scrubbed face of uncertain age, downy and drab with rectitude; the bright eyes, gleaming with fanatic virtue. She comes from nowhere. There is never a car parked on the street that I can see. While I am inside, vacuuming the living room, someone like her has stood at my front door, rung my doorbell and waited with a patient, gladsome smile that insists that the screened door, too, that last filter of domestic privacy, be opened before she states her business.

"We're Jewish," I always say, as she presses her Seventh-Day Adventist pamphlet into my reluctant hands. But she doesn't mind. And by the time I have finished reaching the nozzle blindly under the sofa to pick up dirt that I will never see, and moved the chairs back into their four declivities in the rug, I have almost forgotten her.

"Wait up! Wait up!" she calls, getting closer. There is no escaping her. "I've been chasing you for blocks," she puffs, coming to a stop in front of Peter. "If you don't mind," she announces to me, "I'd like to say a prayer over the child."

I move to stand in front of Pete. I am a wound, a scab, a target, a shield. My mind stings with the shrapnel of moments so awful that they are not like memories at all, but palpable fragments of cruelty, seen, heard and felt again. "Mommy"—a sticky little finger points at Peter in a theater lobby—"what's *wrong* with him?" And Mommy does not answer but drags the child away, head turned over his shoulder, staring boldly, to the safety of some explanation which we do not hear but does not satisfy, and so, again, a whiny "But *why* can't he walk? What's *wrong* with his legs?"

But this woman cannot be dragged away or even stared down.

"Sure," says Peter. "Say a prayer."

I move out of the way.

She places her black-gloved hands lightly on Peter's head and closes her eyes. "Bless this child, O Jesus. Look with mercy and loving kindness upon him and fill him with your healing spirit. Amen." She removes her hands from his head and opens her eyes.

Not too bad, I think; it could have been worse. I smile with relief.

Then she reaches her arms to the sky, her black-gloved fingers stretched and quivering in alleluia, looks into Peter's face and cries out a command: "NOW GET UP AND WALK!"

Before I can kill, before I can stomp her stupid, crazy head into a bloody pulp, Peter speaks: "I'm a little too tired right now. But when I get home and have a rest, I'll try it. If it works, I'll let you know. C'mon, Mommy. Let's go home. I'm hungry."

"Why do they put so many tiny buttons up the back?" Larry complains as he struggles with his thick fingers to fasten the little silk loops around the covered buttons on my wedding gown.

"Probably to make you think twice about getting married. Do up every other one. I just want to find out if it still fits."

"Remember I got hives at our wedding?"

"Remember when Aunt Fanny asked the string quartet to play a *hora*? What a disaster!"

"Do you remember how the wedding announcement read in the *Times* that Sunday?"

"I've forgotten."

" 'Cohen Daughter To Have Nuptials Held.' "

"No wonder I forgot."

"There. You're all buttoned up." I feel his hands sliding around from behind to cup my breasts.

"What are you doing?"

"Holding your nuptials, what else? Turn around. I want to see what you look like."

I look down at the huge white fantasy of a skirt, billowing in soft folds, and try to remember who I was, what I meant, what I hoped. But I can't. All I can see is what I looked like. "The bride will be attired in a gown of white peau de soie styled along princess lines, with Alençon lace fashioning sleeves of elbow length, paneling the front of the bodice and embellishing the front of the skirt, which is draped into a large pouf of peau de soie at the back over fullness that terminates in a chapel train. Her veil is short, secured to a lace-embroidered small crown, and her bouquet is of yellow calla lilies with caladium leaves."

"Come on, turn around," Larry repeats. "I want to see what you look like."

I pick up my skirt, yellowed and crumpled from eighteen years of being stuffed in a box in the attic, and turn around to face him. "I look like Miss Havisham."

He takes a step back. "You look beautiful! It's incredible! Eighteen years and two babies later and your wedding dress fits you perfectly. Maybe it's even a little loose."

Tears rush to my eyes. "It's so much later, so much later. I didn't know . . . It could have been . . ."

"Shhh," Larry covers my mouth gently with his fingers. "There's no point in that. It couldn't have been better; it couldn't have been worse; it couldn't have been any other way than the way it's been."

"But would you have . . ."

"I know. But that's not the point. The point is that we have survived, that we love each other still, that we love each other more. That's what matters. We've been lucky in that. All the rest is talk, so don't," he says, taking his fingers away from my mouth, "say anything but 'I love you.' "

"I love you. I do." I wrap my Alençon lace arms around his neck and kiss him long and soft and sweet on the lips, tasting the tears I didn't know how to cry as a bride.

"I've got to go and give Petie a shower now." I turn and present Larry with a row of buttons to undo. "Release me from this maudlin rig, please."

"I think we ought to try to get away for a few days," he says, starting at the top. "Somewhere warm."

"Oh, Larry, you know we can't. Let's not even talk about it." And then I recite the reasons why, telling them like a rosary. "There's no one to stay with Peter. It's the middle of January, the time when Peter is most likely to catch a cold." I say "*a* cold," even though both of us know I mean "*the* cold."

Positions taken, we each begin to play our accustomed roles.

"We could go somewhere like Sanibel Island so that we could get home quickly if we had to." Larry's voice grows confident, nearly happy with sensed possibilities. "And I bet Pete's special-ed gym teacher . . . Doug—what's his name?"

"Doug Dauz."

"I bet Doug Dauz would be able to stay with the kids at the house. He and Pete are probably on the same school schedule. He can lift Peter and he knows how to piss him, and Pete adores him. I bet if I asked Pete right now with whom he'd rather spend the next five days, Doug or us, I bet he'd pick Doug. Doug's a great guy. He'll do it. I know he will."

"What about Pete? His condition is so perilous. I'm afraid to leave him. Even Sanibel is a long way away. I bet it takes at least six hours. Six hours is a long time. Too long."

"*Six hours?*" Larry's incredulity verges dramatically on outrage. "It doesn't take more than three hours to get to Florida."

"I'm talking door to door." I am a lifer up for parole on good behavior. But I can't take it. I have become my confinement.

"Five hours; six hours at worst. That's enough time to handle an emergency."

"Do you *really* think so? The last time Pete caught a cold, it happened pretty quickly."

"It usually takes a few hours before you can distinguish between a cold and an allergy. The sneezy part takes at least six hours."

"I guess that's how it was last time . . ."

"There are planes at least every hour." Larry seizes the moment. "Why don't I give Doug a call and see if he can do it. Then, if he says yes, we'll work out the other problems. Okay?"

"He's got to promise to call us the first time Peter sneezes, to not even wait for a second—"

"Of course, darling. Hell, it won't be much different than if we went to New York for an evening in terms of getting back. I want us to feel the warm sun. I want us to make love. I want us to sleep through the night. I want us to have fun. Remember fun?" he teases. "That's fun, F-U-N. Since we can't seem to *have* it, couldn't we please *take* it?"

Inside my rib cage I feel a fearful fluttering of possibility, a beating of why not, a soaring of yes. "Yes," I pronounce with a smile, twirling around the room, the peau de soie rustling around me, as heroically determined as Scarlett dressed in the drapes of Tara. "I'll go. Goddamn it, I'll go."

I find that I am not the least bit surprised when the telephone rings. Why not a grade-B fifties setup, something with Van Johnson and June Allyson—a war movie, perhaps:

They've got just a few hours left until oh-four-hundred,

when he has to be back at the base. They've already used up almost half of their time locating a padre. At last they find a room to rent for one night from a sweet old woman who was young once herself. He carries her over their overseas threshold. They kiss. She excuses herself shyly and slips away to change out of her WAC uniform while he prowls the room with a cigarette. She returns in something soft, white and civilian. He puts out his cigarette. And then the telephone rings.

Why not? Life often imitates art; even bad art.

In real life I am unpacking, claiming the top drawer for my underwear, bathing suits and belts, and Larry is removing his tennis racquet, which, he found earlier today, packs perfectly in his suitcase on the diagonal.

"Maybe we shouldn't unpack at all. We might jinx ourselves," Larry is saying, and that is when the telephone rings. Irony is not just a theatrical element. It exists in nature.

"Yes . . . No, I think we'd better not take any chances . . . We should be at the hospital in about six hours . . . Tell them we're on our way."

But it is not until Larry places the receiver back into the cradle that I realize all at once that I have seen this script before, that I have known all along we would have to turn right around and go home.

I knew it when I stuck a push pin in the kitchen bulletin board through *"Mom and Dad's tel. no. in Sanibel";* and when we kissed the kids goodbye, and when I ran back into the house to get my tennis racquet.

"Please, guys, do me a favor. Don't say, 'back so soon,' or 'quick trip,' okay? Your mother is a doo-doo. I forgot my tennis racquet. Goodbye, now!" I wave my racquet in the air. "This time is really Itsville, the final kiss-off. Take good care of each other! Bye guys. Bye Doug."

"Goodbye house, goodbye kids, goodbye driveway, goodbye mailbox . . ." Larry and I call and wave like idiots, backing out of the driveway.

I knew then; a deep, blind knowing. I just didn't realize it. I didn't recognize the feeling. That's why I didn't do anything to stop us.

I knew it when we arrived at the hotel in Sanibel and slung our suitcases on the superfluous second double bed in our room. "We'll unpack later. Let's take a walk on the beach and fit in a swim before dinner."

I knew it when we walked along the beach, heads down, looking for shells and watching our winter-white feet imprint the fine, soft sand near the water's edge.

"Peter wants one of those big conch shells. I think they're found in Florida waters."

"I think they're indigenous to airport boutiques," says Larry. "If we don't find one, we'll buy him one on the way home."

Come to think of it, it's a feeling I've had for months now, an ineluctable pulling sensation—gravid, necessary—like giving in to narcotic sleep. But I didn't realize it until too late, until my head nodded, until the telephone rang and jerked me awake.

"We shouldn't have come. We shouldn't have left him." Larry hangs his head under the harsh sentence.

"Larry, what if it's not of our own making . . . not a matter within our control at all."

"I don't know what you mean," says Larry, snapping his suitcase closed.

"Maybe by turning our backs, by losing control for a moment, maybe we've given Peter the opportunity he's been waiting for . . . a chance to die."

"Take the mask off my face." Peter's voice, soft and breathless, mingles with the vapor under the transparent green plastic, but it is not so muffled that I do not hear him say, "I don't want to spend the last minutes of my life under a mask."

"I can't do that, Petie, I can't," I say, because I can't. After all my years of knowing, after all his years of not

knowing, it is he who can face it. I can barely permit myself
to hear his words, much less follow their brave command.

My hands hang limp and lifeless at my sides, the same vol-
unteering hands that receive their instructions like impulses
from his brain. "Piss me." "Feed me." "Zip me." "Pull my
hat over my ears until the lobes don't stick out." "Turn me
on my side." "Scratch me." My fingers, which by some awe-
some confluence know just where he itches, will not move for
him now.

"You'll breathe more comfortably with it on." That is the
best I can manage, the very best, even though I know that if
he could lift his hands, as lifelike as waxworks, to his face, he
would pull away the mask. I look to Larry, standing across
from me at Peter's bedside. His hands are clenched into fists
at his sides. His face is crumpled with sorrow.

"Take the mask off my face, please," Pete repeats.

I know. We'll negotiate the way we always do. One more
story before bedtime. One more Oreo, just to wash the milk
down.

"I'll take it off for just a moment if you promise to drink
some ginger ale. The doctor said you should drink plenty of
fluids." Games. I am still playing games. Act as if nothing is
happening.

"All right," Peter agrees readily.

"Have we got a deal?" I ask, trying to put a little of the old
lilt in my voice.

"We've got a deal," he says, the way he always says it. It's
all right. Everything is going to be all right.

I bend and gently take the mask between the thumb and
forefinger of my left hand, lifting it out and up, resettling it
on his brow. With the other hand I hold the bottle of ginger
ale and poke the straw between his ready lips. Peter fixes me
with a stern, cold eye and blows.

Bubbles. He blows bubbles. Bubbles of ginger ale build
and billow over the mouth of the bottle, flow down the sides
and over my hand. He is blowing his life away!

"Oh, Peter!" I cry out in pain and pride and joy. "Peter,

you're wonderful. I love you, you marvelous, defiant little sneak. I love you!" I reach down and slide my arms around his body, holding its dead weight against my heart.

"I love you too. And I love you, Daddy," he says, once and for all.

Solemnly Larry reaches behind Peter's neck with his left hand and lifts his head gently off the pillow. His right hand hovers indecisively above the mask on Peter's forehead. My hands tingle and come to life. Quickly I reach for the mask with one hand, release the elastic band which holds it on with the other, and let the mask fall to the floor.

"Thank you," says Peter softly, his voice trailing off as if he were talking in a dream.

We stand at his side, each of us holding a hand, each with a hand on his heart, our fingers laced, listening with our touch to the tiny thump and flutter of his life. Go ahead, Peter, you can die now. Go gentle, darling, go.

His eyes are shut. They twitch like curtains behind which the players are busily taking their places. I can see each vein on the lid, each lash where it meets, enters and disappears, as if the secret of life lay luminous as a tableau beneath that pale, fragile membrane.

The freckles on his nose, splotched and merged by fifteen summers in the sun, seem to fade before my eyes as his skin bleaches to the color of ash.

His lips, still pink and finely delineated by the perfection of innocence, are parted.

I look at his face never to forget, to take it inside me, indelible, still living, to have forever; memorized, but not a memory.

Peter, will you, in death, come and live inside me, never to be born and never to die again, never to become a fading memory: "Was his birthday the second or third of November? How strange, I seem to have forgotten" ... "Was it Peter who said 'Mommy fik-its' or was it you, Adam? Do *you* remember?" . . . "Did he die on February fifteenth, or was it Valentine's Day? Jeezus, Larry, can *you* remember?"

I don't want a fading memory. I want a real, live you, se-
creted inside me. I want to be able to conjure you up, all the
faces of you—laughing, pouting, sticking your tongue out for
a cookie—whenever I want to.

And your voice. I want to hear your voice, I want to have
it. I don't want to have to invent it out of filaments of wispy
recollections, summoned lost chords, stilled vibrations, thin
air.

But that won't happen. I can tell already, just by standing
here, watching, I can tell that you are going away from me.

"Daddy?" Peter's whisper sounds so far away, so lost.
Quickly! I must start memorizing right now. I must get it all
by heart. "Daddy? What does 'impudent' mean?"

Bewildered, frightened, I look to Larry. He answers mat-
ter-of-factly, while tears stream from his eyes, "Impudent. It
means bold. Shamelessly bold."

"Then put me in an impudent position."

Tenderly Larry takes his hand from Peter's heart, takes
Peter's right arm and wraps it around Soft Gray. Then he
looks up at me. I can see from the look in his eyes that he is as
bewildered and frightened as I. Peter isn't making sense.

All at once I understand. He must not be getting enough
oxygen to his brain. "He's hallucinating," I whisper, touching Larry's hand.

No, I can tell. I won't be able to keep you. I can see that
you are going away already. Your words, your breath, are already slipping out of your body, running free, escaping.

See? See that stain of urine growing round and warm on
the starched white sheet? That's death. Oh my God, that's
all there is to it. Just a breakdown of the body, a failure of
the systems, a mechanical event. Funny. I had expected so
much more of death, so much bigger a deal.

I get it now. Now, at the last moment, I get it. It's not for
you I will mourn, who, dying when you were done but not
defeated, died on time.

But what about me? What about me, sentenced for life to
be free of the literal burden of you, yet condemned and ex-

alted to never forgetting. The burden of having you will turn into the burden of missing you.

I won't be able to remember your face! All your living faces will merge into the photograph we will place on the mantel in the living room, and try as I may, soon I will not be able to pull apart a frown from a smile, and little by little I will stop trying and begin to believe that the photo on the mantel is really you because I will have no choice. You will not live inside me. You are going away.

And even after I have unplugged the intercoms, yours from your room, mine from mine, wrapped the brown rubber cord around the white plastic boxes and put them in the attic, will I still hear you calling me in the night, "Mom?," your voice gravelly with sleep?

I suppose I shall. For a while. For a while I will marvel at this macabre, confluent neural circuitry, this phantom pain of a connection that keeps a soldier feeling his amputated leg, that keeps me hearing you.

But soon I will not be able to conjure up your voice, not even your voice telling me that you love me, from the homunculus of you I would, but cannot, sustain within me. Life will not have it. Inevitably, wounds turn into scars, life into memory, or the memory of a memory. That is called healing. It happens in time. They say it is a blessing.

Little will be left, just a permanent soreness and swelling about the heart. But missing you will never heal into a memory. At least I will have that; that and the sad reassurance that it brings, like some fabled time of perfect grace, some Camelot of the spirit, the understanding that I shall never know myself to be so good again.

I feel Peter's heart falter under my fingers—a flutter, like feeling life. Larry clasps my hand. Peter's lips move, and he speaks just one word: "Deliverance." Then the exquisite skin under his eyes twinkles wildly, fracturing like a mosaic, flashing out electric currents as if there were a fire in his brain. His eyes open wide, staring, sightless, yet intent. His head arches back and falls.

ABOUT THE AUTHOR

MARY-LOU WEISMAN grew up in Fairfield, Connecticut, and was educated at Bryn Mawr College and Brandeis University. She has written feature articles for a number of national publications, among them the *New York Times* and *Vogue,* and contributed political and lifestyle satire to a nationally syndicated column, "One Woman's Voice." She teaches writing at Fairfield University and lives in Westport, Connecticut, and Provincetown, Massachusetts, with her husband, Larry, a lawyer. Their son, Adam, is a college student.